MW00475094

Childbirth Choices Today

Childbirth Choices Today

Everything You Need to Know
to Plan a Safe
and Rewarding Birth

Carl Jones

A Citadel Press Book
Published by Carol Publishing Group

Copyright © 1995 by Carl Jones

All rights reserved. No part of this book may be
reproduced in any form, except by a newspaper or
magazine reviewer who wishes to quote brief passages
in connection with a review.

A Citadel Press Book

Published by Carol Publishing Group

Citadel Press is a registered trademark of Carol
Communications, Inc.

Editorial Offices: 600 Madison Avenue,
New York, N.Y. 10022

Sales and Distribution Offices: 120 Enterprise Avenue,
Secaucus, NJ 07094

In Canada: Canadian Manda Group,
One Atlantic Avenue, Suite 105,
Toronto, Ontario M6K 3E7

Queries regarding rights and permissions should be
addressed to Carol Publishing Group, 600 Madison
Avenue, New York, NY 10022

Carol Publishing Group books are available at special
discounts for bulk purchases, sales promotion, fund-
raising, or educational purposes. Special editions can
be created to specifications. For details, contact:
Special Sales Department, Publishing Group, 120
Enterprise Avenue, Secaucus, N.J. 07094

Manufactured in the United States of America

10 9 8 7 6 5 4 3 2 1

Library of Congress Cataloging-in-Publication Data

Jones, Carl.
    Childbirth choices today : everything you need to
know to plan a safe and rewarding birth / by Carl
Jones.
        p.   cm.
    "A Citadel Press book."
    ISBN 0-8065-1640-2
    1. Pregnancy–Popular works.   2. Childbirth
–Popular works.
    I. Title.
    RG525.J673   1995
    618.4–dc20   94-44434
                                           CIP

Contents

4   Obstetric Routines and Procedures   79

5   Cesarean Birth   102

6   Midwifery Care   118

7 Hospital Birth Choices 145

8 Birth in a Childbearing Center 174

9 Birth at Home 198

10   For Us to Create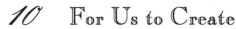   226

Foreword by
Dr. Celeste R. Phillips

This is a book about choice. Its aim is to help you decide the most appropriate way for your child to be born.

For most people childbirth is wellness, not illness. Childbirth marks the beginning not only of an individual but of a family. You owe it to yourself and your baby to consider thoughtfully where you will give birth and how.

Today the childbearing woman has many options. To choose the right health care provider and birthing place for yourself and your family may not be easy. Carl Jones describes contemporary options and presents advantages and disadvantages for you to consider. Talk about the birth options he presents with your partner, family, and health care provider. Ask questions about anything in this book that you want to know more about, and get the answers before making your decision about the place and birth for your baby.

Your birth is just that—yours. It is a special time in your life that you may select for yourself and your partner or share with others you love. Become informed about your options, make safe and appropriate choices, and the birth of your baby will be the happiest day of your life.

Dr. Celeste R. Phillips
Clinical Obstetrical Specialist,
Surgeon General's Office

Foreword by
Dr. Donald Creevy

Where will you give birth? At home, in a birth center, or in a hospital? Or in the birthing bed, on the floor, or in a tub of warm water? Who will attend the birth—a midwife, family physician, or obstetrician? What medical interventions are appropriate? What are safe for you and your baby?

This is a book about choices is childbirth. It is written for all who have an interest in pregnancy and birth—expectant mothers, expectant fathers, siblings-to-be, childbirth educators, midwives, physicians, childbirth companions, and administrators.

As the famous French obstetrician Leboyer gave us a new approach to childbirth in his concept of gentle birth, Carl Jones has given us a new model of labor with his "laboring mind response." His clear description of the laboring mind response—the way the body and mind interact during childbirth—is a breakthrough. It will enable you to understand why guided imagery is such a powerful way to reduce the fear and pain of labor. And it will give you a clear picture of something sadly missing from many childbirth classes, the *experience* of labor—how mind and body interact during labor.

The underlying theme of this book is the inalienable right of parents to choose where, when, how, and with whom they give birth.

Carl Jones never hides his own point of view on any aspect of pregnancy and birth. You always know where he stands: he is the mother's advocate. At the same time he never fails to present a balanced discussion of options. He provides the tools you need to make choices for yourself.

Everyone from the novice lay midwife to the experienced perinatologist agrees that the safety of mother and baby is of the utmost importance in every birth. However, there is widespread disagreement about what constitutes safety in birth and about how the mother can maximize her chances for a safe birth. Carl Jones discusses the alternatives open to each mother and documents his discussion with references from medical literature.

Once you have read this book, you will be equipped to make rational, informed choices for yourself. You will be confident in the knowledge that you have explored each choice to the fullest. You will be prepared to plan the birth that best suits your own personal needs and desires. And most important, you will know how to choose the health care provider and place of birth that is best for you.

Donald Creevy, M.D.
Clinical Assistant Professor of Obstetrics and Gynecology
Stanford University School of Medicine

Acknowledgments

My warmest thanks to my sons Carl (age fourteen) and Paul (age twelve). Together they typed the manuscript and corrected thousands upon thousands of errors, marking places where they felt change was needed. Carl wrote the material he contributed about preparing children for birth (chapter 3) when he was nine years old. His concrete advice is still used today to prepare parents as well as children for the new arrival. At age ten Paul began helping me moderate the worldwide electronic computerized *Birth Forum*, which is influencing the births and parenting decisions of hundreds of people daily.

My special thanks to Cassie Basque, who acted as my research assistant, gathering medical articles as I needed them.

Thanks to the dozens of childbirth professionals who read portions of this book and made numerous suggestions, which helped to improve it.

Those who contributed ideas to the chapter about midwifery care include Joan Remington of the Northern Arizona School of Midwifery; Lorri Walker, certified nurse-midwife, of southern California; Alice Bailes, certified nurse-midwife, of Virginia; and Laurie Foster, a midwife in Vermont.

My wife, Jan, and I both thank Barbara Mason for inviting us to a birth at the wonderful Marchbanks Alternative Birth Center in La Habra, California. This was the first birth—other than her own—that my wife attended.

People who contributed ideas to the chapter about birth in a childbearing center include Barbara Mason; Ruth Watson Lubic of the Maternity Center Association of New York; Karen Knudson of Birthplace in Pittsburg, Pennsylvania; Mary Hammond-Tooke of the Maternity Center in Baltimore, Maryland; Vicky Wolfrum of the South Bay Family Care Center in San Pedro, California; and CharLynn Doughtry of the Labor of Love Childbirth Center in Lakeland, Florida.

Those who contributed suggestions to the section about

xiii

waterbirth include Susanna Napierala, midwife of Glen Ellen, California, and Barbara Harper of Waterbirth International in Santa Barbara, California.

People who contributed suggestions to the chapter about birth in the hospital include Celeste Phillips, clinical obstetrical specialist in the Surgeon General's office; Colleen Gerlach of Birthplace, at Riverside Medical Center in Minneapolis; and many other nurses, midwives, and physicians.

My special thanks to Anne Cleary Sommers, editor of MOM magazine, who encouraged me throughout this project and who spent many hours driving me to childbirth professionals and birth centers when I was conducting workshops in southern California.

I am particularly indebted to the hundreds of parents throughout the United States who have shared their birth experiences with me.

Childbirth Choices Today

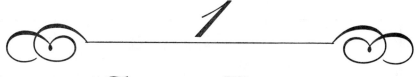

Giving Birth Your Way

Giving birth can be one of the most beautiful and memorable events in your life. The birth of a baby is nature's most awesome miracle. Few things elicit such profound emotions—joy, elation, love. Nothing compares to reaching down and receiving your own child as he or she enters the world, wet and wriggling with life.

In spite of this fact, every year thousands of new mothers leave hospitals frustrated, angry, and sad about their birth experience. Many feel cheated of the joy that a safe, positive birth can offer. One in four mothers in the United States has a cesarean section, though the overwhelming majority of these operations are unnecessary. Many of these cesarean mothers are disappointed, depressed for days, weeks, even months after the surgery. An estimated 60 to 80 percent of American mothers experience some form of "baby blues," a constellation of tears, frustration, and depression beginning sometime during the third to fifth day after birth and lasting from a few days to several weeks—a phenomenon largely the result of unnatural birth customs.

Your birth doesn't have to be this way. You can create the safe, rewarding, joyful birth every parent, every baby deserves.

All parents have different goals and expectations about their birth experience. However, all want a healthy baby, a safe birth, and a positive experience. All parents deserve to enjoy this life-altering adventure to the fullest, and every child deserves to be born into a loving setting.

Fulfilling your own goals is what this book is all about. The chapters ahead and the step-by-step method they outline will better enable you to make well-informed decisions about your baby's

---

What Are Your Options?

You have a variety of contemporary birth options to consider besides conventional hospital labor and delivery. These include

- ◆ Midwife-attended birth in a home, in a childbearing center, or hospital
- ◆ Birth in a homelike setting within a hospital whose staff adjusts their style of maternity care to meet your personal needs
- ◆ Birth in a childbearing center (a place where the mother labors, gives birth, and receives health care during the first postpartum hours)
- ◆ Birth at home

---

birth. They will acquaint you with your choices for a healthy, rewarding birth so you can choose the method that is best for you and your baby. They will provide you the information you need to shape your birth plans and make your birth more rewarding, satisfying, and safer in almost every way.

These are only the basic options. Once you decide with whom and where you want to give birth, your choice should be fine-tuned by a carefully considered birth options plan (discussed in detail in chapter 3) that includes everything from your choice of health care provider during labor to your preferences about obstetrical procedures and routines and your plans for the first days after your child is born.

As prenatal care, better nutrition, antibiotics, and blood transfusions for maternal hemorrhage became widely available over the last few decades, the infant mortality rate dropped. This improvement was paralleled by a higher proportion of mothers who gave birth in hospitals. This connection led to a myth that changed the nation's view of birth: birth in the hospital attended by a physician is safest for all mothers. In reality, no study ever published anywhere in the world at any time in history has ever supported this. In fact, birth in a hospital, in a childbearing center, and at home—though entirely different experiences—are all safe for the healthy mother and baby. The relative safety of each birth option depends on your own health, your health care provider, and your proximity to a backup hospital if a last-minute transfer is necessary.

Whether your birth takes place in a hospital, childbearing center, or at home, you can shape your birth so that it possesses all the following advantages:

◆ Health care during labor tailored to your needs

◆ A philosophy of childbirth in which labor and birth are viewed as a natural, normal process rather than as an illness or clinical procedure

◆ The active participation of the mother in her health care

◆ The active participation of the mother, the father, and possibly the entire family throughout the childbearing process

◆ The recognition that the baby is a conscious participant in the birth process who deserves the most gentle and least traumatic beginning possible to life outside the womb

Childbirth options vary from one area to another. What is considered unusual for one region is the norm for another. For example, in many areas of the United States home birth is not readily accepted and even frowned upon as unsafe, while in the Netherlands—a nation with one of the world's lowest infant mortality rates—home birth is the norm. Likewise, some Americans think of midwife-attended birth as less safe than physician-attended birth, although certified nurses-midwives are licensed to practice in every state in the nation. By contrast, in Japan—the country with the world's lowest infant mortality rate—midwives attend nearly all births. For that matter, according to Dr. Marsden G. Wagner, the European Director of the World Health Organization: "Every single country in the European Region with perinatal and infant mortality rates lower than the United States uses midwives as the principal and only birth attendant for at least 70 percent of all births."[1]

Change in maternity care occurs in response to consumer demand. Certified nurse-midwife Elizabeth Hosford and her husband exemplify the ideal attitude toward making birth choices. They selected a home birth for their first baby over two decades ago. Ms. Hosford writes: "It never occurred to either of us that it was anyone's right but ours to make that decision. . . . It came as a bit of a shock to me in my egocentric pregnancy ecstasy to learn that we were subjects of sharp censure by medical colleagues who assumed it was their prerogative to determine what should happen to us and our baby—and where!

"I felt then as I do now. It is my inalienable right to determine where, with whom, and how I shall bear my children, so long as I do it within the realm of safety. It is up to our Lord to determine when. . . . Freedom of choice with all its implications cannot help but bring a new level of quality to family-centered care. And a new level of optimism across the land."[2]

The Revolution in Childbirth

Fortunately, other parents share the Hosfords' views. A revolution in the way women give birth is taking place throughout the world. Many birth options are becoming more widely available as more parents plan their birth carefully and make well-informed choices about their maternity care.

A more humanized maternity care is part of a major health care trend in which people are rediscovering health care options outside of conventional medicine. An increasing number are turning to such holistic health care methods as chiropractic care, herbal medicine, acupuncture, guided imagery, and other forms of healing—which may be used together with or in place of conventional medicine.

In addition, more health care consumers now take an active role in their health care. Health-conscious people are paying greater attention to nutrition, eating more whole foods rather than the highly processed, chemical-laden foods so common in modern life.

Several other factors have contributed to changes in maternity care. These include dissatisfaction with conventional hospital birth, childbirth education, parents' desire to control the events surrounding the childbearing process, and the parents' need for personalized maternity care.

The women's movement also contributed to an expansion of interest in selecting birth options by making health care consumers aware of their rights in childbearing. A growing number of women

Factors Influencing Changing Maternity Care

- A rediscovery of health care options, from acupuncture to herbalism
- Greater involvement by consumers in their own health care
- Dissatisfaction with dehumanized hospital care
- The women's movement
- Childbirth education
- Education about the laboring mind response (how the mind and body interact during labor)
- The need of parents to take charge of their birth experience

came to desire, if not demand, more involvement in their own gynecologic and obstetric care.

Dissatisfaction with hospital birth grew as parents became aware that it had become dehumanized. Hospital practices were often unnecessary and even inhumane. Mothers were separated from their families and subjected to unpleasant, unnecessary, and sometimes hazardous procedures, from the shaving of pubic hair to the overuse of medications. (Some of these bizarre customs are still practiced in a few hospitals in the United States and Canada.) Laboring women were treated more like invalids than like the healthy women they are.

As their awareness grew, parents gradually became fed up with the customs common in American hospitals. Change was in demand. And change was made. Both the economic threat of losing clients and the discovery of the benefits of more humanized birth helped to make this change.

In response to this dissatisfaction with traditional maternal care, hospitals have made tremendous improvements. In the majority of cases hospital birth is no longer the dehumanizing experience it was. In nearly all hospitals fathers are welcome to attend labors. In the majority mothers and their newborns are not routinely separated. Breastfeeding is encouraged. Yet for the most part, physicians—not parents—still retain control of the events surrounding childbearing, Although this, too, is changing.

Childbirth education has probably played the largest role in revolutionizing childbirth customs. One of the pioneers in this field was the British physician Grantly Dick-Read, who in the 1940s presented a convincing argument against such common obstetric practices as leaving laboring women alone and giving them excessive medication. He stressed the importance of recognizing that psychological factors influenced childbearing. He believed that the pain of labor was the direct result of the mother's fear and tension and that without fear and tension, childbirth would be nearly painless. To decrease fear and tension, he advocated acquainting the mother with the normal process of birth through childbirth education and providing emotional support with the presence of the father or another familiar person during labor. While few agree with Dr. Read's view that childbirth would be painless in the absence of fear and tension, his emphasis on positive changes had a wide influence.

His work contributed to the founding in 1960 of the International Childbirth Education Association (ICEA), a group of childbirth educators. By 1984 ICEA had grown to nearly twelve thousand members in thirty-one countries.

Meanwhile during the 1950s Soviet physicians developed the "psychoprophylactic" method to control fear and pain during labor. The method educated pregnant women about the anatomy and physiology of childbearing and taught them to respond to uterine contractions with patterned breathing and relaxation. It was introduced in France by French physician Ferdinand Lamaze in 1958. An American mother, Marjorie Karmel, who gave birth in Dr. Lamaze's French clinic, founded the American Society for Psychoprophylaxis in Obstetrics (ASPO) in 1960 to teach the Lamaze method. By 1986 there were ten thousand Lamaze instructors in the United States. Though their teaching has been modified several times over the years, many contemporary childbirth educators still consider the Lamaze method mechanistic. Besides, it works for only about 40 percent of laboring women. Hence the method is declining in popularity.

Today patterned breathing (often mistakenly called "Lamaze breathing") is gradually being replaced or combined with guided imagery—a means of translating positive thoughts into dynamic mental images.* What I have termed the "mind over labor" method enables families better to tap their most valuable resource—their inner selves. The method has allowed parents to take more control of their own labor.

During the last couple of decades some forty thousand or more childbirth educators have been certified by ICEA, ASPO, and smaller childbirth education organizations, including Informed Homebirth (IH), the Academy of Certified Childbirth Educators (ACCE), the American Academy of Husband Coached Childbirth (AAHCC), and others. (For more information on these groups, see the Resources section at the end of this book). Though some childbirth educators teach more about birth options than others, most have educated parents to become more active participants in their births.

Many of these childbirth educators are becoming increasingly aware of a phenomenon I call the *laboring mind response*** (discussed in chapter 2). The phrase refers to the psychological and emotional changes that occur during labor—factors more important for the childbirth educator to teach than anatomy. Greater awareness of the laboring mind response continues to contribute to a tremendous expansion of awareness about labor and birth.

Meanwhile such organizations as the International Association for Parents and Professionals for Safe Alternatives in Childbirth (NAPSAC) are helping change childbirth customs by disseminating information about the safety of home birth, midwifery care, and other contemporary options.

Perhaps most important, the desire of parents' to control the events surrounding the childbearing process continues to inspire more changes in maternity care. Hundreds of thousands of parents have discovered they have a right to decide how, when, and with whom they will give birth; in what position the mother will labor; how the father will take part in the childbearing process; and how they will address other concerns of maternity care.

In the 1980s and 1990s thousands of parents became aware

*Though an age-old method, guided imagery was introduced to the American public in the book *Mind Over Labor*.

**I coined the term "laboring mind response" in the *Mind Over Labor Manual*, which is used in workshops to train childbirth educators and other maternity care professionals across the nation. It is currently used in most contemporary childbirth classes.

that the deeply meaningful experience of childbirth had all but lost its unique beauty—physically, psychologically, emotionally, and spiritually—in conventional hospitals. Accordingly, they have chosen to give birth in places where their wishes come before policy, where the love bond between parent and child comes before obstetric protocol, where they have personalized maternity care, where they can be more comfortable, confident, and secure during the childbearing process.

Nothing inspires change more than expectant parents and the choices they make. Every day parents are making fresh discoveries about their birth options. "My first child was born in a hospital," recalls a mother named Beth. "I had epidural anesthesia, numbing and immobilizing the body from the waist down, an episiotomy [a surgical incision to widen the birth outlet], and I gave birth with my legs in stirrups. At the time I thought this was the way childbirth had to be. Later I learned childbirth could be a much different experience. I realized what a total mistake it was to have a baby in a U.S. hospital. My next birth took place at home. I loved staying at home. I didn't have to go anywhere during labor. I didn't have to submit my newborn to strangers. I didn't have to leave my other daughter for two or three days. I felt in control, as if I had really done everything myself."

Not everyone feels this way. In fact, the overwhelming majority of mothers do give birth in hospitals. As birth options become more humanized and widespread, an increasing number have the rewarding experience Beth describes, in and out of hospitals.

Every choice you make, every step you take to shape the birth that is best suited to you will contribute to your health and your baby's.

From the beginning of human life on earth, the birth process has probably remained the same as it is today. However, the way we approach this dramatic rite of passage from womb to parents' waiting arms changes almost daily in one way or another.

Following are some of the latest changes in maternity care:

- ◆ Childbirth centers—facilities in or outside the hospital for prenatal care, labor, birth, and the first hours after birth— have become enormously popular and are now a major industry.
- ◆ Certified nurse-midwives are now legal in every state in the

nation. Many more parents opt for midwives, who, as a general rule, provide more individualized, emotionally supportive care than do the majority of physicians.

◆ Professional labor support providers, called "childbirth companions" or "doulas" (trained to give emotional support and other comfort, such as massage, to laboring women) have become popular throughout the nation. In fact, childbirth companions* have recently made news on national TV, on *The Home Show*, and in the *Wall Street Journal, Newsweek, Cosmopolitan, Glamour* magazine, *Consumer Reports*, the *Los Angeles Times*, the *New York Daily News*, the *Orlando Sentinel*, and elsewhere. Since labor support providers are now available in all fifty states, insurance companies are currently exploring the possibility of underwriting labor companion services to reduce medical costs.

◆ Health care consumers are embracing a wide variety of health care options, including homeopathy, chiropractic care, acupuncture, guided imagery, and many other health modalities. As appropriate, this book will describe these options as well as more conventional medical approaches.

◆ Epidural anesthesia has become much safer and less invasive. In the past an epidural meant complete immobility from the waist down, leaving the mother virtually unable to participate in her own birth. Today a new form of epidural is available, combining an anesthetic agent such as lidocaine with an analgesic such as morphine. The result is pain relief without restricted mobility, and far fewer risks for mother and baby. (Options in epidural anesthesia/analgesia are discussed in detail in chapter 4.)

◆ An increasing number of couples in their thirties and forties are becoming first-time parents. This means a more sophisticated group of consumers, concerned about knowing their options and making well-informed choices.

Childbirth companion, birth companion, and postpartum companion are terms trademarked by the Association of Childbirth Companions (ACC), the organization training and certifying childbirth companions. I founded the ACC in 1993 in response to a need among medical professionals and lay persons to receive professional labor support training.

◆ Expectant parents and others interested in pregnancy, birth, and baby care who have personal computers and modems can now get almost immediate on-line answers to questions from health professionals and communicate with other parents throughout the world via an international forum. (For more information, see Resources at the end of this book.)

Keys to a Safe, Rewarding Birth Experience

Your health and your child's depend largely on healthy prenatal habits and good childbirth preparation. Though you will probably not be able to eliminate all the discomforts of pregnancy and labor, you will increase your chance of enjoying a healthier, happier pregnancy and birth if you observe the following steps:

◆ Get regular prenatal care throughout pregnancy
◆ Eat nutritiously
◆ Exercise regularly
◆ Plan your birth carefully
◆ Meet your emotional needs through labor

PRENATAL CARE

The person who attends your birth—whether physician or midwife—will generally provide prenatal care. It is important to get prenatal care early in pregnancy. Bear in mind, however, that most American women are not acquainted with their birth options until the third trimester. For this reason, it is essential to keep an open mind about your choice of health care provider and be willing to change your health care provider should your desires be better met by another. Be sure to have a copy of your medical records if you change health care providers.

Your first prenatal visit should be a get-acquainted session. Discuss your birth plans (if you have already made a birth option plan) and your feelings about the type of care you would like in labor. Become acquainted with the health care provider's philosophy of childbirth. Some health care providers do not automatically provide routine get-acquainted sessions. State your preferences over the phone when you make your initial appointment.

After the initial consultation, your first prenatal appointment will probably include:

- A complete medical history and physical exam.
- A pelvic exam to confirm pregnancy, to assess the size and shape of the pelvis, to take a Pap smear, and to test for gonorrhea. (Some health care providers wait until the final trimester to do a pelvic exam.)
- A breast examination.
- A weight check so that weight gain can be charted throughout pregnancy.
- A blood test to check blood type and RH factor; to check for anemia, syphilis and other infections, and German measles immunity; and to confirm pregnancy.

Begin prenatal care by the third month of pregnancy to be sure your pregnancy is progressing normally or to spot possible complications.

Attend prenatal appointments with your mate if possible.

During the break at one of my workshops where I had been encouraging childbirth professionals to invite the father to prenatal appointments, a midwife took me aside and said, "I don't just invite them to come, I demand it! I won't even provide care if he is unwilling to attend!"

The father needn't attend every appointment if he doesn't want to, but he should certainly be present at a few. "We thought of our pregnancy as a joint venture," recalls Janet, a new mother. "Kevin attended all prenatals with me; it seemed right for him to share as much as possible."

Attending prenatal appointments together will assist both parents in planning their birth. As Kathy Kangas, mother of three and director of Childbirth Education Services in Worcester County, Massachusetts, recalls, "It was great support to have Tyler at appointments with me. We could both talk about what we wanted. We felt we were creating our birth together."

Though it may mean taking time off work (unless the health care provider has evening hours), the following benefits of father-attended prenatals will more than outweigh the inconvenience or small financial loss:

- ◆ The father is able to evaluate the health care provider and have a part in deciding whether or not to hire this person.
- ◆ He learns more about the pregnancy and becomes more involved.
- ◆ His presence often helps the mother feel more secure, comfortable, and at ease.
- ◆ He can listen to the baby's heartbeat.
- ◆ He can ask questions and air his own concerns.

EATING NUTRITIOUSLY

During pregnancy your nutritional requirements increase over those of the nonpregnant woman in order to meet the needs of your own tissue growth, your increased metabolism, and your developing baby. Eating well is directly related to your baby's well-being and essential to the needs of your changing body. A host of complications can be prevented by observing good nutrition during pregnancy.

Your calorie needs will increase by about three hundred calories daily. Every calorie should count. Avoid empty-calorie junk foods as well as highly processed foods with low nutritional content. Eat healthy snacks between meals, such as raw fruits and vegetables, nuts, raisins, cheese, and granola bars. Cut down on foods like cake, pie, and potato chips.

Your protein needs will also increase. Increased protein intake helps your baby gain weight. Low birth weight has been linked to a variety of complications. Therefore, you should increase your daily servings of such protein sources as meats, fish, and eggs. Vegetarian protein sources include lentils, beans, nut butters, nuts, grains, tofu, and sunflower seeds. If you have a vegetarian source of protein, be sure you are eating a complete protein with all the amino acids. Most vegetarian sources have to be complemented with others; good combinations include rice (preferably brown rice) and lentils; rice and wheat; rice and beans; beans and wheat;

Subsequent prenatal visits will include

- Blood pressure check
- Weight check
- Urinalysis
- Check of uterine growth
- Fetal heartbeat check

---

soybeans, rice, and wheat; and soybeans, sesame, and wheat. It's a good idea to consult a vegetarian cookbook if you plan a vegetarian pregnancy and to discuss your diet with your health care provider.

Your calcium needs will also increase to meet the needs of fetal development and growth of your baby's bones and teeth. You should drink as much as one quart of milk daily or consume its equivalent in the form of cheese, cottage cheese, or yogurt. Other good sources of calcium include tofu, oatmeal, green leafy vegetables, and eggs.

As a result of hormonal change, increased uterine size, and decreased gastrointestinal movement, prenatal constipation is common. To avoid it, include plenty of roughage and fiber in your diet: whole-grain breads and cereals, seeds and nuts, bran (you can add this highly nutritious item to other foods or eat bran muffins if you aren't fond of plain bran), dried or fresh fruit, and raw vegetables with skins and peels on (if appropriate). In addition, drink six to eight glasses of water or other fluids daily.

With a 40 percent or more increase in prenatal blood volume and the baby's storage of iron, you require much more iron than before pregnancy. Iron-deficiency anemia, with symptoms including paleness and feeling tired and weak, may result from inadequate iron in your prenatal diet. Natural iron sources include red meats, liver, egg yolks, blackstrap molasses, and green leafy vegetables. Cooking foods in a cast-iron pan will also increase iron contents, and iron supplements are usually recommended. Some expectant mothers find that these contribute to constipation. However, taking supplements at mealtime with citrus fruit or a glass of orange juice will help alleviate the problem. Folic acid is also often prescribed during pregnancy to prevent anemia. Natural sources of folic acid include liver, brewer's yeast, and green leafy vegetables.

It is best to eliminate alcohol consumption, as alcohol has been associated with abnormalities in fetal growth. The precise limit of safe alcohol intake during pregnancy is unknown. For this reason, many childbirth professionals suggest eliminating all alcoholic beverages during the prenatal months. Others suggest moderation, such as a glass of wine once a week. Check with your health care provider for his or her recommendation.

Everyone these days realizes that smoking is a health hazard, but it poses special problems in pregnancy. It has been linked with underweight babies as well as with an increase in infant mortality. In fact, pregnancy is an ideal time for *both* parents to quit smoking, since even inhaling your partner's smoke is hazardous and can even cause growth retardation. In addition, smoking after birth has been associated with the dreaded sudden infant death syndrome (SIDS). If you must smoke at all after your child is born, be sure your room is well ventilated.

Many physicians fail to stress the importance of a healthy diet with their clients. Obstetricians are taught next to nothing about nutrition during medical school—a peculiar failing of conventional medicine. In fact, most midwives and childbirth educators know far more about nutrition than obstetricians! Oddly, not many years ago obstetricians told pregnant women to restrict weight gain, some even insisting on limiting gain to twenty pounds. This is dangerous advice. There is no "normal" weight gain; it varies from one expectant mother to another. However, an average gain is twenty-four to thirty-five pounds, but up to forty pounds is normal. When I told my seven-year-old boy how some doctors suggest that mothers gain less weight than the combined total shown in the chart below he wrinkled his brow and said, "Don't they teach them math in school?"

Today most childbirth professionals agree that a gain of twenty-four to forty pounds is normal. Some mothers gain more, some less. My wife, Jan, for example, gained only twelve pounds during her first two pregnancies. The pregnancies were perfectly normal, and both babies were in the seven-pound range and quite healthy. But such low weight is the exception rather than the rule—and in fact is usually a cause of concern.

How Your Pregnancy Weight Gain Is Distrubuted

Your baby	7–8 lbs.
Placenta	1–2 lbs.
Amniotic fluid	2 lbs.
Increased breast size	2 lbs.
Increased blood supply	3 lbs.
Retained fluids	3 lbs.
Fat stores	5–9 lbs.
Increased uterine musculature	2 lbs.
Total	25–29 lbs.

Let your body be your guide. Eat balanced, healthy, fully nutritious meals. Ask your health care provider for nutritional information if you are unsure whether or not your diet is adequate.

GETTING REGULAR EXERCISE

Though childbirth is not an athletic event, it is a demanding physical process requiring all your energy. A mother in good physical condition is more likely to have a shorter, more comfortable labor than one in poor shape. Regular exercise will help reduce such common pregnancy discomforts as backache, heartburn, constipation, leg cramps, and fatigue. And keeping fit during pregnancy will enable you to recover your nonpregnant shape more rapidly after the baby is born.

Aerobic exercises that focus on the respiratory and circulatory systems, such as hiking, bicycling, and swimming, are ideal. Many health clubs and gyms have special exercise classes for pregnant women.

Throughout the prenatal months, you are able to do almost everything you could before pregnancy, though your sense of balance is not as good. However, you should avoid beginning unfamiliar strenuous activities and, of course, you should avoid potentially dangerous activities like rock climbing or combat karate! Consult your health care provider for exercise advice tailored to your needs. Ask when in your pregnancy it's best to moderate the amount of exercise.

During our first three pregnancies, regular mountain hiking kept both my wife, Jan, and me in shape and doubtless contributed to her comfortable pregnancy and smooth labor.

Meeting Your Emotional Needs Through Labor

What makes one mother's birth experience an unpleasant event and another mother's a rewarding adventure she remembers with joy? Needless to say, there's no single, easy answer. The health of your baby, whether or not you experience complications during labor, and the degree of discomfort you feel are obviously major factors influencing your birth experience. But in addition to these all-important physical factors, psychological and emotional qualities (such as how you feel about your birth setting or the emotional support you receive during labor) contribute to the birth experience.

Many parents and health professionals don't realize it, but *meeting your emotional needs is just as important for a safe, healthy birth as meeting your physical needs* (see chapter 2).

For example, giving birth in the place where you feel most comfortable and where your emotional as well as physical needs are met can have a profound influence on your labor. It most likely will reduce fear, tension, pain, in some cases the length of labor, and may even influence whether or not you experience complications, including fetal distress and a cesarean section. In addition, your baby can benefit from a gentle, nontraumatic birth in a peaceful setting.

High and Low Risk

Pregnancy is considered high-risk if there are previous medical, current obstetric, or social conditions that are potentially dangerous to the health or life of the mother or baby; for instance, a history of low birth-weight babies, a maternal illness such as diabetes, or a premature onset of labor. Low and high risk, however, are relative terms. Some health professionals are overly stringent in their definition of low risk. For example, some place all mothers over age thirty-five in the high-risk category. However, these women have just as much chance of giving birth normally as anyone else. Every mother—regardless of risk status—can benefit from reading about the options in this book and planning her birth wisely.

If you are considered at risk of developing complications, your options may be more limited than those of the mother with a completely normal pregnancy. You may nevertheless be able to tailor many of the ideas in the chapters ahead to your own situation. For example, in the obstetric department at McMasters University Medical Center in Hamilton, Ontario, Canada, where the latest technological equipment is available for high-risk labors, the mother's children are welcome. A crib or cot is brought into the mother's room so the children can stay with her. A cot is also available for the father or birth partner,* or the father can share the bed with his mate.

Even if you can't find a hospital like this and must give birth in a less than ideal setting, you can still work toward making your birth an emotionally rewarding as well as safe event by looking into midwifery care, hiring a childbirth companion, or making a careful birth options plan.

Summing Up

The birth of a baby is the beginning of a family. As one physician put it, "Birth is a rite of life." It should be just as special as a wedding.

When a child is born, a woman and a man cross the one-way bridge to parenthood. A baby makes the greatest of all rites of passage, from life inside the womb to life in the world. Planning your birth carefully can make that life-altering transition smoother for the entire family. It can make the mother's birth easier and happier. And it can enhance the love bond both parents have with

*I use the term *birth partner* for the father, family member, or friend who gives emotional and physical support to a woman throughout labor. I use the term *childbirth companion* to refer to the professional labor support provider.

their new child. For these reasons, the choices you make now, during pregnancy, can have a long-term positive effect on your entire family.

As more parents learn the value of planning their birth, the options discussed in this book will become more common than conventional hospital birth. When this occurs, glowing birth stories describing labor as a wondrous event will become far more common.

However, the first step begins with learning about the experience—not just the anatomy—of labor.

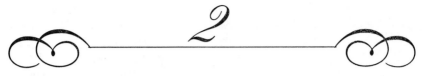

The Experience
of Labor

Understanding the mother's experience of labor is the single most important step you can take toward creating a safer, more fulfilling birth experience. Learning about both the physical and psychological changes that occur as labor progresses will:

- Give you insight into the *experience* of labor, which you cannot get by simply learning about the anatomy and physiology of labor
- Give you insight into the reasons you should plan your birth carefully
- Assist you to make birth plans most conducive to a safe, positive birth experience
- Enable the father or other birth partner to give labor support best suited to the mother's needs

The disappointment many mothers experience in birth can be reduced dramatically by addressing emotional and psychological as well as physical needs. This principle also applies to the baby. We know today that the baby is a conscious and sensitive participant in the childbearing process. Therefore, in planning your birth, you should also consider your baby's emotional as well as physical needs.

A major component is missing from the medical training of most health professionals who assist women through labor: few learn anything about the subjective experience of labor. One cannot learn what the mother experiences by attending medical or

21

midwifery classes, reading texts about the anatomy and physiology of labor, or even acquiring years of clinical experience—though all these steps are necessary in providing competent health care. Being a male in the field of childbirth taught me that the only way to learn about labor is to be with laboring women and absorb what they have to teach through however many hundreds of births it takes. Such learning is not merely cognitive. It requires opening the heart as well as the mind and learning holistically.

Labor consists of a progression of physiological and psychological changes. This observation is the basis of the *Mind Over Labor* method of childbirth I've taught to thousands of childbirth educators. There is really nothing new about this view of labor: midwives have realized for centuries that the mind and emotions influence labor, and labor influences the mind. Mothers have probably always sensed it intuitively.

Nevertheless, a few childbirth educators still teach expectant parents only about the physical process of labor—the changes that take place in the cervix and the physiological mechanism that brings the baby into the world. However, we can no more understand the experience of labor by hearing about cervical dilation than we can get an idea of what lovemaking is like by reading a technical article about tumescence and release in the genital organs.

The mind and emotions influence a wide range of physiological processes from digestion to blood pressure. But of all physical functions, only lovemaking is as readily influenced by the emotions as labor. For this reason, we'll be making some rather striking comparisons between lovemaking and labor.

Since giving birth involves body, mind, and emotions, as labor progresses you are likely to experience profound changes. Your consciousness is altered and passionate emotions are released. Your mind and emotions not only affect whether you have a positive birth experience, they also affect the relative amount of pain you experience in childbearing, the length of your labor, and your baby's well-being.

Whatever factors influence the mind also influence your body. These include your birth environment, your health care provider, the support you receive from your birth partner, others you invite to your birth (from your health care provider to family members), and your own feelings about birth.

The Physical Process

During pregnancy your body prepares for the amazing process that will bring your child into your waiting arms. The *uterus*, shaped like an inverted pear, expands to contain a full one thousand times its prepregnant capacity. Its sturdy muscular walls thicken to keep your baby snug and secure in her temporary home and to push the baby to the world outside when it is time to give birth. The *cervix*—the neck of the uterus which protrudes into the vagina—softens from its cartilaginous consistency (similar to the tip of the nose) to something as soft as an earlobe, *effaces* (thins), and sometimes begins to *dilate* (open) as much as 4 centimeters. By the end of the third trimester, the cervix is *ripe*—that is, partially effaced, dilated, and ready to open a gateway for the baby during labor.

The vagina, whose velvety walls have shaded from a delicate pink to a rich violet during the prenatal months as a result of an increased blood supply, also prepares to stretch. The connective tissue softens and the delicate folds of mucous membrane that make up the vaginal walls prepare to unfold.

During labor, the powerful uterus rhythmically tightens and relaxes. There *contractions* occur intermittently until the baby and *placenta* (afterbirth) are born. Labor contractions are often compared to ocean waves. Each builds, reaches a crest, and ebbs away. At labor's beginning the waves are usually gentle, like little ripples; toward labor's end they may become furiously powerful, like the waves of a stormy sea.

Every labor, like every snowflake, is unique. One mother may labor for two or three days with contractions occurring in an on-and-off pattern, while another may have intense contractions and labor from start to finish in four hours. All labors, however, have three stages.

In *first-stage labor* contractions efface and dilate the cervix until it is wide enough for the baby to be born. Cervical dilation (often spelled *dilatation*) is measured in centimeters (cm). The cervix is said to be fully dilated at approximately ten centimeters (about four inches). As dilation takes place, contractions also push the baby downward so that the cervix begins to stretch over the baby's head like the neck of a tight sweater.

First-stage labor is roughly divided into three phases: In the *latent phase*, or *early labor* (to 4 cm dilation), contractions are usually mild, last from 30 to 45 seconds each, and occur at decreasing intervals from about every twenty to about every five minutes. In the *active phase* (from 4 to 7 cm), contractions may last from 45 to 75 seconds each and occur at decreasing intervals from about every seven to about every two minutes (the average interval being five to three minutes). In *transition* (from 7 to 10 cm), also called late active labor, contractions may last from 60 to 120 seconds and occur at variable intervals ranging from about every three to every two minutes.

The total length of first-stage labor may be anywhere from two or three hours to thirty-six hours or longer. The average duration for first-time mothers is twelve and a half hours. Labor is usually, but not always, shorter for second-time mothers; the average duration for these mothers is about six hours.

Second-stage labor is the birth of the baby. It begins when the cervix is fully dilated. The mother usually feels an urge to bear down and push her baby out. Second-stage may last anywhere from a few minutes to several hours, the average length being one and a half hours for first-time mothers and a half hour for those who have given birth before.

Third-stage labor is the delivery of the placenta. Its average duration is from ten to fifteen minutes.

It's important to know what physical changes to expect during labor. In my opinion, though, preparing for the emotional changes labor triggers is even more important than learning about the mother's bodily changes. After all, the parents don't see the cervix dilate. But they *do* see and experience the laboring mother's altered behavior and altered state of mind.

The information in this summary is based on averages. The length of individual contractions and the duration of each phase may vary widely from the times given here and still be perfectly normal.

The Laboring Mind Response

While the cervix is dilating during first stage labor, the laboring woman experiences a series of dramatic psychological, emotional,

Stages of Labor

Stage/phase	Cervical changes	Length of contractions	Interval between contractions	Duration of stage/phase
First Stage				2–36 hours
Latent phase	cervix effaces and dilates 3 to 5 cm	increasing: 30–35 seconds	decreasing: 20–5 minutes	6–8 hours
Active phase	cervix dilates from 3–5 to 7–8 cm	increasing: 45–75 seconds	decreasing: 7–2 minutes (average 5 to 3 minutes)	2–3 hours
Transition phase	cervix dilates from 7 to 8–10 cm	increasing: 60–120 seconds	variable: 3–2 minutes	½–2 hours
Second Stage	birth of baby	6 seconds	variable: 5–2 minutes	a few minutes to 2 or more hours
Third Stage	delivery of placenta	variable	variable	10–20 minutes

and behavioral changes. Taken together these make up what I call the *laboring mind response*.

The idea came to me while I was giving workshops to childbirth professionals and heard many describe how difficult it was to teach parents about these aspects of labor. I developed the concept of the laboring mind response for two reasons.

First, I wanted to give expectant parents and childbirth professionals a description of the *experience* of labor, rather than merely the physical process. My goal was to convey—in simple, down-to-earth language—the laboring woman's altered state of mind, as well as the psychological and behavioral changes that occur as labor progresses.

Second, I wanted to explain why, in simple terms, guided imagery was such an effective means of reducing the fear and pain

---

The Laboring Mind Response

As labor progresses, most all women experience the following seven characteristics to a greater or lesser degree:

◆ Greater right brain hemisphere orientation.

◆ An altered state of consciousness.

◆ Altered perceptions of space and time.

◆ Heightened emotional sensitivity.

◆ Decreased inhibitions.

◆ Distinctly sexual behavior.

◆ Greater openness to suggestion.

---

of labor. Any childbirth professional who has tried the method realizes that guided imagery is more effective than patterned breathing for relaxation and pain reduction, yet few could explain *why* this is so.

The laboring mind response consists of seven characteristics that most women experience to a greater or lesser degree. The father (or other birth partner), as well as the mother, should learn about these characteristics in order to better understand his mate's experience and provide effective labor support, thus reducing the mother's fear and pain. For this reason, I will show how the seven steps apply to the birth partner.

1. The right brain–hemisphere becomes more dominant. As labor progresses, the focus of the laboring woman's energy seems to shift from the left hemisphere of the brain to the right. The left hemisphere is associated with logic, reasoning, analytical thinking. The right hemisphere (sometimes called the heart brain), on the other hand, is associated with creative and artistic thinking, intuition, lovemaking, and labor. As the right hemisphere comes to dominate the scene, the mother becomes more intuitive, emotional, and instinctive.

The birth partner who is aware of the laboring woman's right hemisphere orientation will be better able to provide the emotional support and encouragement the mother needs. He will understand, for example, why giving her emotional support is often more effective than giving her a series of instructions (though instructions may at times be helpful).

2. *The laboring woman experiences an altered state of mind.* The mother may greet labor's onset with any of a wide variety of reactions. She may be anxious, elated, relieved, excited, talkative, and so forth. Regardless of these responses, if contractions are still mild, she may be able to function pretty much as she always does, continuing with her everyday life or going back to sleep if it is night.

Once labor is under way and contractions continue to dilate the cervix, however, she experiences a profound psychological transformation. Her consciousness is altered—as if the contractions that are opening the cervix were also opening a primal part of her mind.

Along with her greater right hemisphere orientation, the mother becomes less rational, more instinctive, and more intuitive. She seems to enter her own world. As one father put it, "It was as if she were in a different world, traveling in a new dimension as she lay in my arms." Expressing a similar idea, Dr. Richard B. Stewart of the Birthing Center at Douglas General Hospital in Douglasville, Georgia, says, "If you provide the proper environment, a laboring woman will go into her own psyche and shut out the external world."

As a result of this temporarily altered consciousness, many mothers forget to do things they have planned. For example, the mother may forget something she has learned in childbirth class about coping with contractions, or a mother who plans to view the birth in a mirror may forget all about this when the time comes. Her birth partner can help by reminding her to do what she has planned, *if* she still wants to do it.

The laboring mother's concentration narrows and she becomes more introspective, or inner-focused. Her contractions and those persons in her immediate environment become her world. The birth partner's presence, love, and support will assist the mother to yield to the psychological changes labor triggers and thereby experience a less painful and more efficient labor.

One new mother told me, "I never understood what you

meant by the laboring mother's altered state of mind until I was in labor. Then it all made sense to me!" This is true of many women. The mother—to say nothing of the father—often has no clear picture of labor until she is actually experiencing it.

3. *The laboring woman experiences altered perceptions of space and time.* As labor moves along, the mother's perceptions of space and time seem to become progressively distorted. For example, laboring women frequently think contractions are lasting longer than they actually are.

The laboring mother becomes wholly caught up with the forces that are bringing her child into the world. Odd as it may sound, some women may even lose sight of the fact that they are going to have a baby! It is as if, in her profoundly altered mind, she forgets the purpose of what she is experiencing. The birth partner can occasionally remind her she will soon see her baby.

4. *The laboring woman experiences heightened emotional sensitivity.* As labor progresses, the laboring woman becomes highly sensitive, vulnerable, and dependent on her birth partner and those around her. Almost all mothers experience this heightened sensitivity, particularly toward the end of first-stage labor.

At the same time, the mother's emotions influence her labor. Every parent and childbirth professional should be aware of this connection. A disturbance in the environment can cause labor to slow down. It is well known, for instance, that contractions often slow down and sometimes peter out altogether when the mother enters the hospital. Presumably this is because the mother is anxious in the unfamiliar environment.

The birth partner who is aware of the profound impact emotions have on labor will be able to reduce significantly the mother's fear and pain by being an emotionally nurturing and supportive presence.

5. *The laboring woman usually has lowered inhibitions.* Social inhibitions tend to be dramatically reduced during the course of labor. This is an individual matter. Some women become less uninhibited than others. A few always remain self-conscious of what others may think of their behavior. But the majority become remarkably unconcerned.

The laboring woman may remove all of her clothing as labor nears its end. She may groan, moan, and sigh like a woman nearing sexual climax, though she feels nothing like it! She often becomes unconcerned with who sees her unclothed body or hears the sensual sounds she makes. This behavior is especially common at a home or a childbearing center because the alternative setting is usually most conducive to a normal and spontaneous reaction to labor.

The birth partner should realize that this relaxing of inhibitions is normal, to be encouraged. It is a sign that the laboring mind response has been elicited.

6. *The laboring woman exhibits distinctly sexual behavior.* Lovemaking and labor are obviously poles apart. Sex is associated with pleasure and labor with pain. However, since both labor and lovemaking take place within the sexual organs, labor is a sexual process. This does not mean that labor is a sexual experience, or necessarily pleasurable.

There are striking similarities between the two processes. The following list is based on my own observations of laboring women, combined with those previously noted by other childbirth professionals.[1]

- ◆ During both labor and lovemaking, the uterus rhythmically contracts, though the contractions are far more intense during labor.
- ◆ During both processes, the vagina lubricates and opens.
- ◆ Both processes are associated with the right hemisphere of the brain.
- ◆ During both labor and lovemaking, a woman becomes intensely emotional and vulnerable.
- ◆ Emotions influence both processes. Disturbances, emotional conflicts, and inhibitions can impair both.
- ◆ Social inhibitions decrease during both labor and lovemaking.
- ◆ A woman has a similar expression—something I think of as a tortured/ecstatic look—near sexual climax and toward the end of labor.

- During both processes women often make similar sounds—moaning, sighing, groaning.

- Both processes are often followed by a state of well-being.

- Both are primal processes that are most satisfying when a woman surrenders body, mind, and emotions to the experience.

Surrendering to labor, letting go, yielding to the experience is the key to a smoother, less painful, and more rewarding birth experience. To put it another way, the same conditions that are conducive to satisfying lovemaking are conducive to a safe, positive birth experience. These include peace, privacy, comfort, subdued lighting, freedom from disturbances, and the ability to surrender to the process and to react spontaneously.

Surrendering to the amazing changes of the laboring mind response is the key to letting labor work in the most efficient way. This doesn't mean you can't distract yourself from pain if necessary by concentrating on a focal point, regulating your breathing, or using guided imagery. Rather, it means you should accept as normal the psychological and emotional changes labor precipitates.

Understanding this characteristic of the laboring mind response will enable the birth partner to relate better to the mother's behavior. For example, he should be aware that groaning, sighing, and moaning are a normal reaction to labor for some, but not all, women. Some misinterpret the mother's sighing and groaning as signs of pain. Though these sounds may be reactions to pain, they do not necessarily indicate pain. The sensual sounds the mother makes are part of the natural voice of the laboring woman. They well up from the soul. Accepting this behavior as normal will assist the mother to surrender more easily to labor.

I often point out how the vagina lubricates and opens during both labor and lovemaking. Labor also triggers a psychological as well as physiological opening. "You want to open for your baby like you open for your lover," I suggest to women in my workshops. This lovely metaphor elicits an almost visceral reaction.

Laboring women appear to sense the need to open on a deep, intuitive level. The very word *open* has almost magical power during active labor. Using a soft, soothing voice to tell the mother to think of herself opening and perhaps at the same time imagine the cervix dilating—like a blossoming flower—can often cause a difficult labor to progress more rapidly.

7. *The laboring woman experiences an increased openness to suggestion.* During active labor the laboring woman becomes more easily influenced by suggestion than perhaps at any other time in her ordinary waking life. She enters what I think of as a quasi-hypnotic state, where suggestion has great impact. For example, a health care provider, impatient for labor to be under way, enters the room and says, "Your labor is progressing awfully slowly." Though such a simple suggestion would probably have little or no effect during ordinary waking life, once the laboring mind response has been elicited, the suggestion may actually cause the mother's contractions to slow down.

Toward the end of labor, suggestions seem to have a magnified impact on the woman. The good news is that this applies to positive as well as negative suggestions. Such comments as "You are really doing fine!" or "You can do it!" can help the mother better cope with labor. Likewise, the positive suggestions of guided imagery can have a powerful effect on helping her through labor. The birth partner should be as positive as possible in his words and actions.

Anticipating the laboring mind response will help you and your mate to plan a more rewarding childbearing experience. For example, if you recognize that labor triggers profound emotional and psychological changes, you will be likely to choose a physician or midwife with whom you feel psychologically compatible. With the mistaken assumption that medical competence is the only important factor, the majority of pregnant women put little thought into their choice of health care provider. This misunderstanding leads to many disappointing birth experiences. You have a far greater chance of a positive birth if you select a health care provider who understands your emotional as well as physical needs, or who at least respects your individual goals regarding childbearing.

Similarly, you will also see the need to select an emotionally positive birthing environment where you are free to surrender to the laboring mind response. Maternal and infant health and the fulfillment of the mother's emotional needs are inextricably linked.

The birth partner—as well as the maternity care professional—who is familiar with the laboring woman's behavioral changes and heightened emotional needs will be better able to provide effective labor support. For example, he will see why caressing her and giving her verbal encouragement in a soft, soothing voice is often more effective than "coaching" her with regulated breathing. Above all, he will recognize that the most powerful support he can give is his love.

Developing a Positive View of Birth

A positive view of birth is the cornerstone for preparing for a safe, rewarding childbirth experience. The mother who believes that her body was designed to give birth normally is more likely to have a smooth labor than the woman who believes that giving birth is a potential disaster. In my opinion there are four key components to a positive image of birth. I have taught thousands of maternity care professionals to use these key components as assessment tools to evaluate whether or not their client has a positive view. You can use them as guidelines to assess your own beliefs.

1. *Childbirth is a normal healthy event, not an illness.* No one, of course, actually thinks that childbirth is an illness. However, many parents and professionals *act* as if it were.

The fact that birth is unconsciously linked with images of disease is one of the major reasons hospital birth is so much more common than out-of-hospital birth in the United States. In America the laboring mother is often cast in an invalid role, as if she were helpless and in need of hospitalization. This peculiar custom has affected the birth experiences of millions of mothers. Educating parents and professionals about other contemporary birth options begins with believing that birth was designed to be a healthy, normal process.

2. *Birth is a natural process, not a medical event.* Though it sounds absurd to remind anyone that birth is natural, this seemingly obvious fact needs to be reinforced—particularly in the United States and Canada, with their over 25 percent cesarean rate and high rate of obstetrical intervention. For many parents and profes-sionals, childbirth conjures up images of women with IVs, elec-

tronic fetal monitors, and other medical equipment. While medical intervention is sometimes necessary, today, with our emphasis on medical technology, we often lose sight of the birth process itself.

Appreciating that birth is a natural process doesn't necessarily mean that the mother is committed to laboring and giving birth with no medication (though this is almost always safer for her and her child). Rather it implies that she accept that birth, like conception, is a physiologically natural process.

3. *Childbirth is a social event.* Birth is the beginning of a family and is one of the most significant social transformations in the lives of most couples. Labor is an awesome rite of passage for the entire family. The baby makes the dramatic passage from life inside the uterus to life in the world. A man and woman cross the one-way bridge to parenthood. A child becomes a brother or sister.

I often encourage parents to think of their birth as they would their wedding. You should make it just as special, just as beautiful.

4. *You, the parents, are the center of the childbearing drama.* The mother *gives* birth. It is her strength and power that brings her child into the world, and it is the birth partner's support that enables her to release this strength and power. The birth partner's strength consists of giving the mother nurturing emotional and physical support throughout her labor. In addition, the parents are the center of the childbearing drama in that they, not the medical staff around them, should be in charge. This is one of the many points that distinguishes a rewarding birth from one that leaves the mother feeling cheated and deprived of something essential. When she is treated as the center of the childbearing drama, she is often less tense and is able to react more spontaneously to labor and therefore labor more smoothly, her mind and body working in harmony.

Reducing the Pain of Labor

The degree of pain in labor varies from one woman to another. A few women experience almost no pain, but most find labor hard and painful work. As one mother put it: "It was difficult but never more than I could bear."

Labor is not continuously painful. The mother experiences the most discomfort during contractions, and the pain of contractions varies throughout labor. Generally speaking, contractions that occur toward the end of first stage labor are considerably more painful than those at the beginning.

Second stage labor usually feels quite different from first. It can vary widely, from intensely difficult to exquisitely pleasurable. For some mothers, the actual birth process is as painful as the first stage, if not more so. For most, however, the second stage is less painful. In one mother's words: "It was incredibly exciting! The pain of contractions left when the cervix was fully dilated."

Third-stage contractions are often barely noticed in the excitement of holding the new baby.

The pain of labor is different from other kinds of pain you may have experienced. Many have described it as "positive" pain, a contradictory-sounding expression that seems to refer to two things. First, labor contractions are purposeful; the pain is "healthy" pain. Each contraction brings the mother a little closer to seeing her baby. At the same time, the powerful contractions of late first-stage labor massage the baby and prepare her for her first breath. Second, though it is painful at times, many mothers find labor a rewarding, fulfilling experience, something no one would say about a toothache!

Giving birth in a setting where your emotional as well as physical needs are met can dramatically reduce the pain of labor and heighten your joy in birth. In addition, the two most effective non-pharmacological means of reducing the fear and pain of labor are the support of a nurturing mate or other birth partner or childbirth companion and the use of guided imagery, a technique that is now taught in most childbirth classes. For some, breathing patterns, particularly when combined with guided imagery, can be helpful.

Bear in mind that labor is not all pain. Labor encompasses a wide variety of feelings from agony to ecstasy. If it were solely an unpleasant experience, we would not hear so many new mothers, radiant with joy, exclaim, "I want to do it again!"

THE LAMAZE METHOD

The Lamaze method, also called the psychoprophylactic method, was introduced by French obstetrician Ferdinand Lamaze. This method provides knowledge of the anatomy and physiology of labor to help the expectant mother overcome fear, relaxation practice to diminish tension and pain during contractions, and breathing patterns to be used as an aid to relaxation or a distraction during contractions. Today, the label "Lamaze" covers a wide variety of childbirth classes, some of which have almost nothing in common.

Most Lamaze instructors teach patterned breathing. Hundreds of Lamaze childbirth educators have learned about the benefits of guided imagery and are teaching this in place of, or in addition to, the breathing.

PATTERNED BREATHING

In the past most childbirth educators taught patterned breathing, and this method of coping with labor is still widely taught. Breathing patterns are intended to help the laboring woman relax and cope with contractions and to distract her from the pain. Patterns include

◆ *Slow breathing,* to be used when contractions are mild

◆ *Accelerated or light breathing,* to be used when contractions are more difficult

◆ *Pant-blow* breathing, to be used when contractions are at their most difficult

Breathing patterns help only about 40 percent of laboring women reduce the fear and pain of labor. If you are attracted to the method, combine it with guided imagery to make it more effective. I don't teach health professionals breathing patterns for a number of reasons. For many mothers, breathing patterns interfere with a spontaneous response to labor and can actually impede labor's progress. Also, fathers frequently become so involved in helping their mates with patterned breathing that they lose sight of what are more effective means of labor support, like whispering encouraging words or hugging the laboring woman. If your educator teaches breathing patterns, think of them as backup, to be used when and if you have the need.

THE MIND OVER LABOR METHOD

This method of childbirth preparation and coping with labor is based on understanding the laboring mind response, making birth plans tailored to your individual physical and emotional needs, and using guided imagery.

Guided imagery (sometimes called *visualization*) is an excercise whereby a person translates positive thoughts into dynamic mental pictures or images. You can use it for a number of goals, including reducing tension, fear, and pain; developing confidence in your ability to cope with labor; making better birth plans; and enhancing prenatal bonding and your sense of communication with your unborn child.

Guided imagery has been used in healing for centuries. The method has begun to spark the enthusiasm of professionals the world over, and today guided imagery is used with great success in a wide variety of fields including medicine, psychotherapy, education, business management, stress management, and sports training and competition. It is also effective for childbirth.

While only some mothers find relief during labor in patterned breathing, all can benefit from using guided imagery either by itself or in addition to breathing patterns. Emmett Miller, M.D., world pioneer in the field of psychophysiological (mind-body) medicine, has found that the method can reduce the need for pain-relief medication and for obstetric intervention, including the use of forceps.

Many women don't realize how effective guided imagery is until they are actually in labor and the laboring mind response has been elicited. For example, one woman told me that at first she didn't like the exercises I taught because they didn't offer the discipline of Lamaze breathing. When she was in active labor, however, the breathing patterns she had learned in childbirth classes and practiced during pregnancy did not reduce her tension and pain. That was when she began using the guided imagery exercises. After a beautiful, natural birth, she exclaimed, "I never thought guided imagery would be helpful. But that's what got me through labor!"

Why Does Guided Imagery Work?

Guided imagery is ideally suited to the expectant and laboring mother for two reasons.

In the first place, guided imagery is a right-hemisphere process, and the mother experiences greater right brain–hemisphere orientation both during pregnancy and especially, as we have seen, during labor. Since you are more right hemisphere–oriented during labor, the method is probably more effective in labor than at any other time in your ordinary waking life. According to Dr. Miller, guided imagery translates cognitive information into terms that can activate the right hemisphere and actually help bring about an easier, more fulfilling labor.

In addition, guided imagery gives you strong positive suggestions at a time when you are wide open to suggestion. To make the method even more effective, you can combine guided imagery with affirmations or strong positive statements such as "I am able to give birth in harmony with nature" and "I trust my body to labor smoothly and efficiently."

Benefits of Using Guided Imagery

During pregnancy, guided imagery

- Promotes relaxation of body and mind
- Develops the mother's confidence in her ability to give birth safely and positively
- Develops the father's confidence in the birth process and in his ability to give effective labor support
- Enhances prenatal bonding
- Helps both parents make better birth plans
- Reduces the likelihood of postpartum blues

During labor, guided imagery
- Helps the mother relax
- Reduces fear
- Reduces pain
- Reduces in many cases the length of labor
- Reduces the likelihood of complications, including fetal distress and cesarean section
- Helps the parents create a safe, positive birth experience

If your childbirth educator does not cover guided imagery thoroughly in your classes, see the book *Mind Over Labor* for the dozens of relaxation and guided imagery exercises you can use during pregnancy, labor, and breastfeeding.

COMBINING GUIDED IMAGERY AND PATTERNED BREATHING

Any breathing method works well with any guided imagery exercise, though it is best to breathe deeply and rhythmically while doing imagery exercises. Here are some specific suggestions for combining these two coping methods:

- Use *The Opening Flower* during late labor, imagining the flower blossoming on the breath out.
- Use *The Radiant Breath* imagery during contractions. Imagine the radiant light travelling with the breath to the area of discomfort or tension and massaging the pain or tension away with its soft, golden radiance.

LABOR IN THE WATER

Many women find it soothing to sit in a tub of warm water during active labor. For this reason an increasing number of hospitals and birthing centers now include bathtubs, hot tubs, Jacuzzis, or whirlpools on the maternity unit. The mother usually labors in the tub, then gets out sometime before it is time to give birth, though some give birth in the water.

Cindy, a mother from Indiana, recalls, "I'm not usually one for long baths but I must have spent half my labor in the bathtub! Nothing seemed to soothe me like the hot bath. My husband, Gary, spent most of the time pouring water over my abdomen and wondering when I'd be out of the tub."

Many health professionals advise expectant mothers to avoid tub baths once membranes have ruptured. When the amniotic sac has broken, there is a risk that bacteria may enter the uterus and cause infection. However, immersion in water is acceptable once the mother is in active labor, since there is no time for an infection to develop.

"When labor is in progress," points out Dr. Michael Rosenthal of the Family Birthing Center in Upland, California, "everything is headed downstream, inhibiting the passage of bacteria up the birth canal into the uterus, even if there were time to develop an infection."

As ridiculous as it sounds, in a few hospitals mothers are not allowed to use the Jacuzzi once membranes have ruptured. The Jacuzzi is used only during early labor, which is unfortunate since it is during late active labor that the mother will most benefit from immersion in warm water. Once after lecturing at a hospital where a Jacuzzi had recently been installed, I asked a nurse if she thought it was helpful to laboring mothers."Women hardly ever get to use it," she said with obvious vexation about her hospital's policies. Fortunately, that policy was changed.

A hot tub bath with the water as deep as possible can be particularly relaxing when contractions mount in late first-stage labor. In addition, immersion in a hot bath can facilitate labor's progress, assisting the mother to have a more efficient labor.

Researchers at the University of Copenhagen, Denmark, compared a group of laboring women who bathed in a hot tub bath for a half hour to an hour with another group of laboring women who did not use the tub. They found the laboring women who spent time in the bath experienced pain relief as well as more rapid cervical dilation (2.5 cm per hour in the bath group compared to 1.26 cm per hour in the nonbathing group).

Water may assist the mother to labor more efficiently in a number of ways. In his March 1990 article, "Birth in the Water," which appeared in the prestigious British medical journal, The Lancet, Dr. Michael Odent writes, "We believe that the warm pool facilitates the first stage of labor because of the reduction of the secretion of catecholamines [stress hormones]; the reduction of sensory stimulation when the ears are under water; the reduction of the effects of gravity; the alteration of nervous conduction; the direct muscular stretching action; and peripheral vascular action."

Dawn, a mother who gave birth in a tank of warm water in Maidstone Hospital in Kent, England, recalls, "The tank was still being filled and the water was not at the required depth. Nevertheless, all I wanted to do was strip off and jump in, and that is exactly what I did."

A hot shower can also be relaxing. The mother can stand under the shower and let the water play over her back and abdomen.

I recommend the birth partner help the mother bathe or shower. While the mother is taking a bath, the father can pour water from a glass or pitcher over her abdomen if she finds this helpful. If she is showering, he can stand nearby or shower with her if he prefers. He can bring swim trunks along if the mother is laboring in a hospital or childbearing center.

Hot compresses can also promote relaxation and ease pain during labor. The birth partner or health care provider can wet a hot towel and wring out excess water, then apply it to the area of discomfort, such as the lower back or abdomen. The compresses should be changed often to keep them warm.

Waterbirth

If the mother chooses to give birth in the water, she remains in the tub throughout the birth process and sometimes for a short while afterward. The heath care provider can monitor the labor's progress and the baby's heart tones in the water just as on a labor bed.

Dr. Robert Doughton, who has assisted with nearly one hundred waterbirths in Portland, Oregon, points out that warm water contributes to perineal relaxation. "Nothing can better relax the perineum than a body-temperature bath," he says.

In addition, as Dr. Odent points out, "Immersion in water seems to help women lose their inhibitions." Losing her inhibitions can enable the mother to surrender to labor and thereby give birth more efficiently.

Most mothers deliver in the sit-squat position or on hands and knees. Providing the tank is large enough, the mother is readily able to adopt the position of her choice. One mother squatted with her husband's support as she pushed. When the baby's head was crowning, she sat back in the water to give birth.

The physician, midwife, and nurses usually remain outside the tub where they can assist if necessary. If the tub is sufficiently large, the mother's mate and perhaps others can join her. For example, one couple, Nancy and Gaston, remained together in the pool. The midwife got in when Nancy was close to giving birth.

Immediately after birth, the baby is lifted slowly and gently to the surface. She may open her eyes and look around, unfurling her limbs, while still under water. Once at the surface, the newborn's breathing is triggered by contact with the air and by the sudden difference in temperature and pressure.

The parents can begin the process of parent-infant bonding in the tub. The mother can hold her child to her breast and begin breastfeeding or just explore her child with her eyes and fingertips. The father too can hold the baby skin-to-skin and enjoy eye contact in the tub.

The baby's body is kept warm in the water. With her mother's or father's hands on her back for support, the baby can lie back and float.

Erika recalls, "After Jason was born, I held him so his face was above water and let him float for about twenty minutes." When it was time for third-stage labor (the delivery of the placenta), Erika got out of the water and delivered the placenta while semireclining on a bed near the insulated water tank she had used.

To avoid potentially serious complications, it is best to get out of the tub to deliver the placenta. It's difficult to monitor the volume of blood loss in the water, and the process can be rather messy, since the mother may lose considerable blood with the afterbirth.

Many women find that waterbirth creates an easier, less painful, and shorter second-stage labor. As one mother put it, "I think the delivery was significantly less painful than it would have been on land. I was also able to spread out my energy consumption more easily. I didn't tire myself out."[2]

Convinced of the benefits of waterbirth, pioneer obstetrician Michael Rosenthal assists mothers with waterbirth at his Family Birthing Center in Upland, California. More waterbirths have occurred there than anywhere else in the United States. In March 1990 the center celebrated its six-hundredth waterbirth out of the nearly two thousand births since it opened in 1985.

Because the Family Birthing Center is one of the few centers in North America where waterbirth is an option, women travel from as far as Alaska and Montreal to give birth there. Two warm-water baths measuring six feet long by four feet wide by eighteen inches deep are available for laboring women.

Other childbearing centers throughout the world are beginning to include waterbirth. For example, the Natural Childbirth Institute and Women's Health Center in Culver City, California, has had about a dozen waterbirths over the past few months. The midwives plan to see more women use their newly installed tub for waterbirth. Nearly three hundred babies have been born in the water at St. James Natural Childbirth Clinic in Malta. Almost a hundred waterbirths have occurred in Federal Hospital in Oberpullendorf, Austria. Other hospitals, such as Maidstone Hospital in Kent, England, are just beginning to learn about waterbirth and to accept it as a safe alternative.

Waterbirth is attracting an increasing number of parents, and advocates for this childbirth option are increasing yearly. An organization called Waterbirth International (WBI), was founded by Barbara Harper, RN, in Santa Barbara, California, in 1989 to provide information, referrals, videotapes, tub rentals, seminars, consultations, and prenatal classes for parents and professionals interested in waterbirth. WBI's goal is, as Barbara Harper puts it, "To turn the tide on the current high-tech, hospital, medically controlled approach to childbirth back to family-centered birth, where the intuition of the birthing woman is respected and the baby is included as a conscious participant in its own birth."

Speaking of waterbirth at Pithiviers, Dr. Michael Odent observes, "We have found no risk attached either to labor or to birth under water." After his experience with over six hundred waterbirths at the Family Birthing Center, Dr. Rosenthal says he has seen no complications.

The two problems parents and professionals are most concerned about are the mother developing an infection and the infant inhaling water with a possible risk of pneumonia or drowning. There is very little risk of infection to the mother, provided the water is clean, and waterbirth advocates agree that there is virtually no danger of the newborn drowning, if the baby is taken to the surface immediately after birth.

Dr. Odent says, "To this day, we have never needed to clear breathing passages after such a birth, nor have we had minor infections or complications associated with underwater births."[3] Dr. Odent adds· "Women seem to know that it is not at all dangerous to give birth in water; there is no risk to the newborn, who, after all, has known only watery environments."[4]

For a short while the infant continues to receive oxygen through the umbilical cord. The baby does not actually begin breathing on her own until reaching the air. As Dr. Rosenthal points out, "Within seconds after the birth, the placenta begins to separate from the uterine wall because the amount of uterine wall surface has been enormously reduced and the placenta is not elastic enough to remain attached. . . . the oxygenation of the fetal blood that is being brought to the placenta decreases immediately."[5]

In an article in the *Journal of Nurse-Midwifery*, Linda Church, a midwife from the Family Birthing Center in Upland, adds, "Although the infant goes from one watery environment to another and does not take its first breath until its skin thermoreceptors are stimulated by air contact, it has minimal oxygen reserves. Because the placenta ceases to function as completely as before—even with a pulsating cord—once born, the infant is on its own and must be immediately lifted to the air to breathe."[6]

The Newborn Bath

Immersing the baby in warm water immediately after birth, many parents and professionals believe, significantly reduces trauma. The "Leboyer bath," or postnatal warm-water bath, was popularized by the well-known French obstetrician Frederick Leboyer, who advocated a gentle birth process.

Dr. Leboyer's concept of gentle birth consists of several practical steps. First, birth should take place in a quiet place with subdued light. After nine months in the womb, the baby's eyes are quite sensitive. If the room is brightly lit, the baby will screw up her eyes to shut out the light. If the lights are subdued, however, parents and baby can enjoy that wonderful experience of eye contact that follows a natural birth. Second, keeping the environment free of unnecessary noise prevents the baby from being rudely shocked after having heard only muted sounds in the womb.

Immediately following birth, parents and baby should be together for the bonding process for at least one hour without interruption. All newborn procedures, such as the use of eye drops to prevent infection, weighing, measuring, and the routine newborn exam, should be delayed. Unless there is a medical reason to do otherwise, the umbilical cord should be allowed to finish pulsing before it is cut. This way the baby receives the additional blood still in the placenta. Once the cord is cut, Dr. Leboyer advocates placing the baby in water which has been heated to body temperature. There, in the warm-water bath, the baby will open her eyes and calmly take in the environment, gazing at her parents' faces.

Today the Leboyer bath is commonplace in hospitals throughout the United States.

Interestingly, when the Leboyer bath was first introduced in the United States, professionals had a concern about safety similar to the one they now have about waterbirth. Strict sterile technique was employed, including a sterilized stainless steel basin and sterile water for the bath. Now, however, these unnecessary procedures are no longer observed. Professionals have learned that heated tap water is perfectly fine.

There is little doubt that the newborn bath can reduce postbirth trauma, particularly in the clinical environment of the stainless steel delivery room. Trauma, however, is probably better minimized by choosing a suitable place for a child to be born. You can create a gentle birth, whether or not you use a newborn bath, by giving birth in a dimly lit, homelike environment and delaying all newborn procedures for at least one hour. The best place for the baby during the first postnatal hour is at her mother's breast or held skin-to-skin against father's chest, not in a tub of water.

It is important to realize that gentle birth has far-reaching implications and may actually be the beginning of a nonviolent life. After a lengthy investigation of the "roots of crime," the Commission on Crime Control and Violence Prevention in Sacramento, California, recommended, among other things, childbirth with parental involvement, family intimacy, and a natural delivery that discourages overuse of intensive-care nurseries and labor-inducing drugs.

Midwife Anne Rivers agrees. "For me, waterbirth is more than just a comfortable way to birth a baby. Consciously creating peace for our children from the very moment of birth is the gentle beginning of new possible harmony."[7]

The Childbirth Companion

"When I was in labor with my daughter Chelsea," recalls Jacki Elledge, a massage therapist and childbirth companion, "it was a nightmare of fear and confusion. As labor waxed intense, I forgot everything I had practiced in childbirth classes, everything I had read. No one was there to support my husband, Clay, and me. As nurses came and left the room, they told me I was doing great. At what, I wondered? Panicking?

"Months after Chelsea was born, I observed a labor attended by a childbirth companion—a person specially trained to give emotional support. There was something special about this birth. The mother worked with her labor with a sense of contentment that I'd never before seen on the face of a laboring woman. And after the birth, the baby had a peaceful look about her, like she was glad to be here."

Jackie now works as a childbirth companion, giving families experienced support and encouragement. With a childbirth companion at their side, they no longer have to experience the confusion and fear she and her husband felt.

"Every woman should consider having a professional support person," asserts John Kennell, M.D., of Case Western Reserve in Cleveland, Ohio.

These unique childbirth professionals are called a variety of peculiar names, including "monatrice," "coach," and "doula," none of which actually describes what the childbirth companion does.

How Parents Benefit

In a recent American Medical Association study, Dr. Kennell showed that the presence of a trained childbirth support person cut the cesarean rate to less than half, decreased the need for drugs, reduced pain, and led to significantly shorter labors and healthier babies.[8]

With such methods as guided imagery, childbirth companions are skilled in helping the mother reduce pain and relax. They are taught to manage difficult labors, help prevent unnecessary cesareans, provide breast-feeding support, and support the father so he can better participate in the birth of his child.

In many birth settings the childbirth companion is the only person who remains with the parents throughout labor and the early postpartum period. Most physicians are present only during the final part of labor to assist during the birth. As a general rule, midwives remain with the laboring mother for a longer time but not throughout her entire labor. In most hospitals nurses come and go as the shifts change. The childbirth companion, on the other hand, is a familiar face from the beginning to the end of the mother's labor.

The childbirth companion can offer perspective, reassurance, encouragement, and suggestions. She is an invaluable assistant to VBAC (vaginal birth after cesarean) mothers, single mothers, and others who simply want the presence of another knowledgeable person besides their health care provider.

Courtney, a new mother, can vouch for the benefits of a childbirth companion from personal experience. "Without Lori, my childbirth companion," she recalls, "I'm sure labor would have done me in, as the expression goes. During many hard-to-handle contractions, Lori was indispensable to me. Her soothing voice, caring smile, and warm supporting arms meant the difference between manageable contractions and being dominated by pain."

"We were·a team," recalls Courtney's husband, Bill. "Lori worked with us through it all. She helped Courtney keep her breathing relaxed and easy, gave her relaxing guided imagery exercises that reduced her pain, and took turns with me giving back massage. She even applied warm compresses to the perineum (area between anus and vagina), which prevented Courtney from tearing, saving her weeks of discomfort."

Cheri, a new mother, recalls: "We wanted a childbirth companion for a couple of reasons. First, in case we had to transfer to the hospital, I felt it was important to have someone present who understood our needs. I didn't want my husband, Martin, to run interference for me through labor. Second, I wanted him to be at my side the whole time, completely focused on me and not to have to leave for anything. Kathy, my childbirth companion, did lots of odd jobs like keeping the Crock-Pot warm and so on."

Kristi Ridd, a childbirth companion in Salt Lake City who has attended over two hundred births, says, "When I work in a hospital setting, I help couples understand their choices in maternity care and help them make informed decisions. So many adults have been taught never to question the health care professionals. It's okay to ask questions and important to make one's own choices."

Physicians who have had the chance to observe childbirth companions are beginning to write prescriptions for their clients so that the childbirth companion's services are covered by insurance.

Hospitals and birth centers are beginning to hire childbirth companions. For example, the Washington Birthing Center in Fremont, California, has childbirth companions on call around the clock. According to Dr. John Kennell, childbirth companions may spell multibillion-dollar savings to maternity hospitals on epidural anesthesia, cesarean surgery, and other costly medical procedures. "We calculated that on the four million births per year, there could be more than two billion dollars a year in savings if every mother had a childbirth companion."

Childbirth companions are usually nurses, midwives in training, childbirth educators, or laypersons. Most have special training and experience in giving labor support as well as assistance during the early postpartum period. Though a medical background is not necessary, the childbirth companion must complete the requirements established by the Association of Childbirth Companions (ACC), the national organization that certifies and regulates childbirth support providers. Certification involves a three-day training program, hands-on experience at a birth, and required reading of books and medical articles.

There's a reward for the childbirth companion in addition to the $250 to $500 per birth she takes home. As Carolyn, a Nevada childbirth companion, puts it, "I can offer loving and nurturing support while receiving so much gratification!"

"The hours are long, the work is hard, and I must always be on call," says Judy, another childbirth companion. "But the joy and thrill of welcoming a new life envelops me every time I attend a birth. I feel as if a part of me is reborn with each birth. When I attend a birth, I'm not just a helping professional. I share the mother and father's feelings, their fears, their doubts, their disappointments, their triumphs, and their joys.

"I'm there not only to give support but to share a miracle!"

CHOOSING YOUR CHILDBIRTH COMPANION

Here are some guidelines for hiring a childbirth companion:

- Interview the childbirth companion to be sure the person is someone with whom *both* parents get along.
- Be sure your childbirth companion is fully supportive of your birth plans.
- Find out what assistance she offers. Is her role limited to

giving labor support? Or does she also help out during the early postpartum period?

Many fathers prefer to be the sole and primary support person, with no one else present during labor. For other couples, however, the childbirth companion can enhance the father's ability to give effective support in the way that is most comfortable for him.

Looking Ahead

The experience of labor can be be defined in terms of how the cervix dilates and how the baby descends in the birth canal, yet you must also take into account your psychological and emotional changes and how these influence the physical process. There is more to giving birth than the observable realities of hard science. Labor affects the mother's whole being—her mind and emotions— as well as her body. Realizing this is, in my opinion, the key to shaping a rewarding birth experience you'll always remember with joy.

In the past, conventional obstetrics, by focusing on the physical experience alone, has robbed the birth experience of its beauty and individuality. Childbirth education is changing this as more educators learn about and teach the psychological and emotional changes described above. Throughout the world, an increasing number of health professionals are teaching the laboring mind response. Though I've explained some of the psychological aspects of labor in terms of the laboring mind response, there is yet another facet of labor that cannot be reduced to a formula, seen on a monitor, or measured in a laboratory. That is the essential mystery of labor. We can describe the physiological changes. We can approximate in words the psychological and emotional changes the laboring woman experiences. But can we explain what takes place when what was a tiny seed no larger than the head of a pin makes the awesome rite of passage to become "my son" or "my daughter"? That is something a parent must experience to know.

In my opinion, adopting a new model of childbirth based on understanding the psychological as well as physical process of labor is the most significant step we can take toward a safer, saner obstetrics.

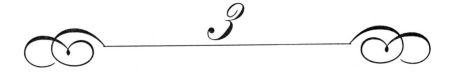

Planning Your Birth

Creating a birth options plan* carefully will help you reduce the fear and pain of labor; have a safer, more fulfilling birth; and enjoy healthier, less stressful days after the baby is born. If you have a choice, create your birth options plan during the early months of your pregnancy. Unfortunately, few parents do so. Many, if not most, first-time expectant parents don't learn about all available childbirth options until late in pregnancy. This is one reason you should keep an open mind until you are sure your birth plans are the best you can make. Also, many parents don't realize the value of creating a birth options plan until after a disappointing birth experience, often involving an insensitive health care provider or an unnecessary cesarean.

Every mother—regardless of her risk status—can benefit from planning her birth with care. An essentially healthy mother whose pregnancy has little chance of medical complications is considered low-risk. If you are low-risk, you can choose from any of the options in this book.

Since there are so many options available, it is essential to make choices carefully. For example, the majority of women who have had joyful, rewarding birth experiences in or out of the hospital have read a book like this, taken childbirth classes, and discussed their options with childbirth professionals and other parents. For the most part, they are better informed than most

*The birth options plan in this chapter is adapted from *The Childbirth Companion*—the training manual used to educate professional labor and support providers. It is now taught in many childbirth classes throughout the world.

The Benefits of Planning Your Birth

Planning your birth carefully can help you achieve:

- An emotionally positive climate for birth
- A more efficient, more comfortable labor
- Freedom of mobility throughout labor
- Freedom to labor and give birth in the position of your choice
- Freedom to breathe and push in harmony with your body's needs
- Freedom to eat and drink to satisfy your needs
- Less need to use pain medication
- Avoidance of unnecessary medical intervention

---

mothers who give birth without first visiting several hospitals or interviewing health care providers.

With the *laboring mind response* in mind (see chapter 2), you can see how drawing up a careful birth plan can alter your birth experience tremendously.

Choosing or Assessing Your Childbirth Class

Now that you have a glimpse of the *laboring mind response*, you are already on your way to preparing for a safe, rewarding birth and reducing the fear and pain of labor. One step toward these goals is choosing your childbirth class (or assessing your present class) with great care.

Good childbirth classes provide you with an opportunity to learn about labor and your options regarding birth, to air your concerns, and to meet other expectant parents who probably share many of your feelings.

Your childbirth educator can play a vital role in preparing you and your birth partner for a safe, positive birth. She (the overwhelming majority are women) can give you a clear idea of what to expect in labor, acquaint you with your choices in

---

Essential Elements of a Birth Options Plan

- Choosing a health care provider
- Choosing health care options
- Planning the role of the father or other birth partner
- Choosing your baby's health care provider
- Deciding who will attend the birth (siblings, relatives, friends, childbirth companion)
- Choosing a childbirth class
- Preparing for labor
- Arranging for help at home after birth

---

childbirth, teach effective ways to cope with labor, and help you tailor your birth experience to your individual needs.

Nevertheless, many parents leave childbirth classes without having learned about *any* of these topics. For this reason, you should interview a childbirth educator and find out what she teaches. Find out your childbirth educator's opinion about electronic fetal monitors, intravenous feeding, episiotomy, and all medical procedures and obstetrical routines. Many instructors don't teach the disadvantages as well as the advantages of medical interventions during labor. In fact, many don't know this information themselves. If you have not interviewed your educator carefully before signing up for classes, do so now, even if classes are in midstream. It is better to educate yourself than to take a class that does not cover all the topics discussed ahead. Why? Because a class that fails to cover these topics can leave you with misinformation, doing far more harm than good.

When my wife and I learned we were going to have our first child, we, like many foolish consumers, signed up for childbirth classes without interviewing the teacher. During the first class the instructor assumed that all her clients were planning a hospital birth without asking if some might prefer to give birth in other surroundings. We never went back to that class.

Following is a checklist of things to ask yourself and your educator about your childbirth classes.

◆ *Does your childbirth educator leave you with a clear picture of the psychological dimensions of labor?* Does she teach the laboring mind response or all its characteristics under another name? "I was totally unprepared for labor!" exclaimed one new mother who had taken eight weeks of childbirth classes. "The instructor taught tons of breathing exercises but didn't give me the slightest idea of what labor would be like." I hear this kind of comment all the time. Your educator should be well aware of the laboring mind response. Be sure she is covering this information.

◆ *Does your childbirth educator place hospital, childbearing center, and home birth on an equal footing?* You want to select the birth place with which you are most comfortable. Acquainting parents with their birth options is an integral part of good childbirth education, and every childbirth educator is obligated to cover all these choices. Many educators, however, discuss only hospital birth. While hospital birth may suit the needs of many parents, it is not for everyone.

◆ *Does your childbirth educator inform you about the pros and cons of all medical procedures and obstetrical routines?* Rather than give the parents the information they need to make well-informed decisions, instructors all too frequently prepare the mother to be a compliant patient who will accept hospital policies and medical routines without question. At one class I observed, an instructor held up an amni-hook (something that looks like a crochet needle) and said, "This is what will be used to break the waters." She never suggested that some women might not want their waters (amniotic sac) broken.

◆ *Does your childbirth educator encourage you to create a birth plan to meet your own individual needs?* Ideally, you will be able to find a childbirth class that will help you clarify and achieve your goals for the birth you desire.

◆ *Does your childbirth educator prepare the birth partner for his support-giving role?* The childbirth educator who understands the laboring mind response will encourage the father to be nurturing, to maintain physical closeness with his mate, and to be emotionally supportive. In addition she will teach him a wide variety of comfort measures, such as massage for back pain. In the past some child-birth educators referred to the father as the "labor coach"—a term that gives him a wholly inappropriate view of his role in labor. The coach belongs on the football field, not in the birthing room. Some women like their birth partner to give them instructions; this, however, does not make him a "coach." The term can have a negative impact on the father in two ways. First, it encourages him to dominate and control the mother's reactions to labor—the very approach that should be avoided. Second, it distances him from the childbearing miracle. Being a coach is much like being behind a camera, instead of being part of the event.

◆ *Does your childbirth educator cover guided imagery, not just patterned breathing?* In all the years I've lectured to thousands of mothers and maternity care professionals, I have yet to meet the woman who did not find guided imagery a more helpful tool than patterned breathing. Some women find that the two methods work well in harmony. However, all find guided imagery helpful in a wide variety of ways.

◆ *Are your classes small—with no more than ten couples?* You will receive far more individualized attention in a class with six to ten couples than in a class of thirty.

◆ *Are your classes held on neutral ground (in a private home or church, for example)?* These are usually preferable to those sponsored by a hospital. Though many hospital classes are excellent, most do not encourage mothers to learn about alternatives and to take an active role in their own health care.

◆ *Do your classes support breastfeeding rather than put breast and bottle feeding on an equal footing?* The health benefits for your child of breastfeeding are superior to formula in every way. If your childbirth educator does not make this clear, she is doing your family a disservice.

◆ *Do your childbirth classes cover information about preventing unnecessary cesarean sections?* If your classes merely present facts about cesarean surgery without giving tips on how to avoid a cesarean, they are incomplete.

◆ *Do your classes inspire both parents' confidence in their ability to handle labor*—the mother's confidence in her strength and power and the father's confidence in his ability to give effective labor support? Both parents should receive encouragement.

If the answer to more than one of these is no, take a good, hard look at your class. Vital information is missing. A class that does not cover all of the above can do more harm than good. If you have more than two *no* answers, seek another instructor. If you can't find an educator who meets these standards in your area, consider educating yourselves. You can use the self-taught curriculum in the Appendix at the end of this book, and if you have access to a computer with a modem, you can get on-line help from *Birth Forum*. Information about connecting with *Birth Forum* is included in the Resources at the end of this book.

Choosing or Assessing a Health Care Provider

Several kinds of health professionals besides midwives and obstetricians provide maternity care. These include family practitioners, naturopaths (physicians specializing in natural healing methods), and in some areas, chiropractors. When I use the term *health care provider*, I am encompassing all these professionals.

Whether physician or midwife or other, a good health care provider is a guardian of a natural process, present to assist when needed and to intervene only if necessary. This definition is based on the philosophy that birth is a natural process, not a medical event. Keep this idea in mind when selecting the person who will help you at your birth.

All of the suggestions to follow apply whether you are meeting a health care provider for the first time or assessing your current health care provider. If you are already seeing a health care provider, assess this person in the light of your newly acquired knowledge and be willing to change if necessary. The single most common reason women complain of difficult, even harrowing birth experiences is a poor choice of health care provider. Be sure your mate reads this section. It cannot be repeated too often. Read the preceding two paragraphs again (aloud if necessary) until you believe them. The integrity of your birth depends on this vital choice.

The most important thing to look for in your choice of health care provider is, of course, medical competence. Be sure the person who gives prenatal care and who attends your birth is able to handle an emergency should one arise.

- ◆ *Interview your health care provider.* You are hiring a professional to attend an extremely intimate event. As Kristi Ridd, national coordinator of the Association of Childbirth Companions, puts it, "You should choose a health care provider for birth as carefully as you would select a lover. Anything less is cheating yourself."

- ◆ *Ask relevant questions.* For instance, Amy, a Detroit mother, was planning to give birth at home. The first thing she asked was how many home births her health care provider had attended. She then asked what equipment the health care provider brings to the home. Sara, a New Hampshire first-time mother, wanted to avoid an episiotomy. The first question she asked her doctor was his episiotomy rate. When he replied, "I do episiotomies on most first-time mothers because I feel they are necessary," she politely left his office.

- ◆ *Meet the assistant or backup physician as well.* Most midwives and some physicians will work with an assistant. There is much to do during labor and an assistant's hands are usually needed. Some health care providers work in a group practice. Meet every member of the health care team.

- ◆ *Select a health care provider with whom you feel psychologically comfortable.* After all, you are inviting this person to share one of the most intimate events of your life. You want to share it with someone you like and whose philosophy of childbirth is close to your own. *Both* parents should feel reasonably compatible with the health care provider. If the father is uncomfortable with the midwife or physician, this may diminish his own experience of the birth. In addition, if he's uneasy, this will be communicated to his mate and make her uneasy as well. For example, Karen and Mark, a couple in Maine, changed health care providers because their midwife had a strong prejudice against male birth attendants. "She said she believed the father's place was at his mate's side during labor and had no problem with fathers at birth," Mark recalls. "But her anti-male attitude seemed to color her entire practice. I didn't feel right paying someone a fee who had this kind of problem with men in her profession."

Of course, in some areas, like the rural area where I live, your choices may be limited. But if you do have several options, make your decision with great care.

MIDWIFE OR PHYSICIAN?

Many expectant parents feel most comfortable with a midwife at birth. Others prefer an obstetrician or family practitioner.

Actually, you can have both. The midwife-physician team is an ideal birth attendant partnership. The midwife provides care for healthy pregnant and laboring women. The physician is present in case complications arise.

In some areas a certified nurse-midwife (CNM) attends home births. The CNM is trained in a hospital setting and typically has much experience. However, this background can give some CNMs an overly clinical view of birth.

The well-trained direct-entry midwife (one who is trained through a midwifery school and/or apprenticeship) can be a highly competent birth attendant. Many midwives who are trained through a combination of apprenticeship and midwifery school view birth as a natural process rather than a medical procedure. However, if you choose a direct-entry midwife, it is imperative that she (or he) be highly qualified (see chapter 6).

MALE OR FEMALE?

After a workshop where I had been describing how labor affects the mind as well as the body, a midwife turned in an evaluation with the following comment: "I can't believe it! I never realized a man could actually understand labor!"

Many people—childbirth professionals as well as laypersons—believe that women make better nurses, midwives, childbirth companions, and primary health care providers than men. This is just like the old-fashioned prejudice that kept women from medical school. The qualities of the health care provider are what count, not the gender.

I also once thought that a woman—by virtue of having given birth—would have greater insight into the labor experience and be more sensitive to another woman's needs than a man. Experiences at scores of births, however, have taught me this isn't so. The fact is that men can be just as sensitive and nurturing as women at birth. Likewise, there are insensitive health care providers among both sexes. So have an open mind when choosing your health care provider.

Selecting a Birth Place

Whether you give birth in a hospital, childbearing center, or home, it is essential to choose the birth environment carefully. Never make your selection based on such factors as insurance coverage.

Visit several birth places before making a final choice, even if you have already selected. As professor of obstetrics at Stanford University, Don Creevy, puts it, "The person who selects a hospital without visiting it is an even more foolish consumer than the person who buys a home over the telephone."

You will be more likely to have a safe, positive birth in a place you feel provides an emotionally positive climate. The safety of the birth environment is, of course, the prime concern for most mothers. Some parents think this means having medical equipment available. While available equipment is certainly a factor in a safe place of birth, an emotionally positive climate also contribute to safety. The birth environment can influence uterine function, the length of labor, how much discomfort the laboring woman experiences, parent-infant bonding after birth, and even whether or not the mother develops complications.

Laboring in a nonclinical environment with an emotionally positive climate can lead to a more efficient labor. This is because the physiology of labor, like that of lovemaking, is influenced by emotions and can be affected by disturbances in the environment.

It is well known that labor often slows down and sometimes

even stops entirely when the mother enters the hospital, presumably because of the mother's anxiety in the unfamiliar environment. As Dr. Stanley Sagov, Dr. Richard Feinbloom, and their associates point out in their text *Home Birth: A Practitioner's Guide to Birth Outside the Hospital,* "Some women may react to the stresses of the hospital environment by developing tensions that in turn complicate labor and may therefore require medical interventions that would not have been required in their homes."[1]

A similar argument can be used to justify hospital birth if that is where the mother *feels* most comfortable. In fact, some women's labors don't get going *until* they are in the hospital. According to certified nurse-midwife (CNM) Ruth Watson Lubic, founder of the Childbearing Center in New York, during the first year the center was opened, many mothers did not progress in labor until they were transferred to a hospital, again presumably because they were anxious in the unfamiliar setting.

In an eye-opening study, Dr. Niles Newton, former professor in the department of psychiatry at Northwestern University, found that disturbances in the environment had a significant health impact on laboring mice. A number of mice near delivery were moved every hour or two from a familiar sheltered cage to a glass bowl with cat odor, so that an equal number of mice were always in both bowl or cage. A far greater number of mice delivered in the sheltered cage. In a similar study with laboring mice, researchers found that disturbances contributed to a 65 to 72 percent delay in labor.[2]

Selecting Health Care Options

When you plan your birth, you will find it helpful to draw up a written health care checklist as part of your *birth options plan.* The purpose of a checklist is to:

◆ *Inform your health care provider of your plans* so he or she can meet your individual needs. It's a tool to communicate your plans and preferences to anyone giving prenatal care, attending your birth, or providing baby care.

◆ *Make you more aware of your options and clarify your preferences* regarding important details of obstetrical and pediatric care during labor, birth, and the early postpartum period.

♦ *Help you make contingency plans* for the unexpected, such as a transfer from home to hospital, a cesarean section, or unforeseen emergencies. If a transfer from home to hospital must be made during labor or if a cesarean section unexpectedly becomes necessary, both parents are bound to be overwhelmed. Making the contingency plans *now* can help you avoid much anxiety and the need to make decisions at the last minute.

Discuss the items on the list with your health care provider and ask to have a copy of the list included in your chart. You may want to ask your health care provider to sign the checklist, giving his or her approval of your preferences. Make copies of your checklist for your health care provider, the person providing backup care, and your baby's health care provider. This will enhance your chance of having the birth experience you planned for.

The shorter, more concise, and more flexible your *health care checklist*, the more likely your health professionals will take it seriously. Remember, your *list* is a communication tool, not something that should elicit antagonism.

Note: All expectant parents deserve to be able to create the birth they desire and have *all* their preferences honored, whether giving birth at home, at a childbearing center, or in a hospital. Unfortunately, however, many parents are not able to have everything they want, depending largely on the hospitals and health care practitioners in the area where they live. Unless you are willing to go to great lengths to fulfill your goals (such as temporarily relocating), you may have to be flexible about some details.

Following are some suggested items to include on your *health care checklist*, based on the recommendations of the Association of Childbirth Companions. The details reflect the personal preferences of hundreds of well-informed parents who have planned their births after thoroughly researching their options. You can use this as a base to create your own birth options plan, if you wish. Or, depending on your own personal preferences, you can create an entirely different set of options.

SAMPLE HEALTH CARE CHECKLIST

For Labor and Birth

◆ The father (or birth partner) and you are free to remain together without separation for any reason.

◆ Your invited guests—siblings, family, friends, and childbirth companion—are free to remain with the parents through labor and/or birth as the parents choose.

◆ If you are planning a home birth and should there be a transfer from home to hospital, the home birth midwife is free to remain with you throughout hospital admission, labor, and birth.

◆ An electronic fetal monitor is to be used only if there are signs of fetal distress.

◆ Use of an IV for intravenous feeding is to be reserved for emergencies.

◆ Only a minimum of internal exams are to be performed.

◆ No pain relief medication is to be offered unless you request it.

◆ No episiotomy is to be cut unless there is a clear case of fetal distress, shoulder *dystocia* (difficulty delivering shoulder), or other medical emergency requiring a surgical incision.

◆ You are free to take a shower and bathe whether or not membranes have ruptured.

◆ You are free to drink fluids and eat lightly as you wish.

◆ You are free to walk around during labor.

◆ You are free to labor and give birth in the position of your choice.

◆ Labor and birth are to take place in the same room.

◆ You are free to reach down and complete the delivery as soon as the head and shoulders are born.

◆ Your mate is free to catch the baby or assist during the birth as he wishes.

◆ Your mate is allowed to cut the umbilical cord.

◆ You are free to deliver the placenta spontaneously without uterine stimulants.

For the Immediate Postpartum Period:

◆ You and your baby are to remain together without interruption for at least one hour, unless there is a life-threatening medical emergency requiring immediate pediatric attention.

◆ You are free to dim the lights to enhance early parent-infant eye contact.

◆ You are allowed to breastfeed immediately after giving birth.

◆ The use of eye drops to prevent infection and the administration of the vitamin K shot are to be delayed for at least one hour following birth.

◆ Routine baby care procedures, such as weighing, measuring, and footprinting, are to be delayed for at least one hour following birth.

◆ All baby care—including the newborn exam—is to take place in your presence.

◆ If you give birth in a hospital or you are transferred to one, no bottles of formula or water are to be given to the baby at any time during your stay.

◆ Siblings and other family members are allowed to greet the baby face-to-face within the first hours after birth.

◆ If birth takes place in a hospital, you and your baby are allowed twenty-four-hour rooming-in.

◆ Your mate is free to remain with you and your baby twenty-four hours a day.

◆ You and your baby are discharged twelve to twenty-four hours after birth, unless there are medical complications.

For Cesarean Birth:

◆ Your mate is free to remain with you throughout surgery and preferably throughout preoperative procedures.

◆ You are given options regarding type of anesthesia.

◆ You decide whether or not to take any preoperative or postoperative medications.

◆ Your mate may hold the baby close to you immediately after birth, unless there are life-threatening complications requiring immediate pediatric attention.

◆ You have one or both hands free (rather than strapped to the operating table) to caress your child.

◆ Your mate is free to accompany your child to the intensive care nursery if there is a medical emergency requiring immediate pediatric attention.

◆ Your mate is free to remain with you in the recovery room.

◆ You and your baby remain in the same room for twenty-four hours. Your baby is never removed from you for any reason other than a dire pediatric emergency.

◆ Your mate may remain with you throughout your postpartum hospital stay, twenty-four hours a day.

◆ No bottles of formula or water are to be given to your baby at any time during the hospital stay. The baby is breastfed exclusively.

◆ You are discharged within forty-eight hours if you wish to go home and your condition warrants it.

Planning for the Father's Role

The father can participate in childbearing in a wide variety of ways, from just observing the birth to "catching" the baby as he or she is born.

As I see it, the father's *primary* role during labor is to experience the birth of his own child. At the same time, he can reduce his mate's fear and pain tremendously and make her feel more confident, secure, and comfortable. There is no right or wrong way for the father to be involved. He should take on whatever role is comfortable for him and his mate.

Some fathers simply want to be present while another family member, a friend, or childbirth companion gives active labor support. "I asked other people for support with the breathing and relaxing," recalls Jean, who has had one hospital and three home births. "Tony didn't feel comfortable doing all that. He just wanted to be there. And that was really the best thing for me, just to have him with me and know that someone else was taking care of whatever else needed to be done."

Other fathers want to give the primary labor support. If the father chooses to do this, he may want another family member, friend, or professional childbirth companion present to give backup support. Regardless of the role he elects to take on, every father should be thoroughly familiar with effective ways of reducing his mate's fear and pain.

Some fathers want to catch their own child. This can be a wonderful experience. If the father decides to do this, the health care provider usually assists with the delivery of the baby's head, that part of birth most in need of expert assistance. Then the father can complete the delivery. As the baby is born, the mother can reach down, take the child under the arms, and bring her to her breast.

Whatever role the father assumes, I suggest he cut the umbilical cord. The bluish white cord is curly, like the receiver wire of a telephone. One end is attached to the baby and the other to the placenta inside the mother, but cutting it does not hurt either mother or baby. The cord will continue pulsing for a while after birth, as blood passes from the placenta to the baby. Clamping and cutting should be delayed until the pulsing ceases, unless there is a medical reason for doing otherwise. The birth attendant will first prepare the cord by clamping it on either side of the place where it is to be cut. The cord is then cut with a pair of scissors. I think of cord cutting as a dramatic ritual concluding childbirth's rite of passage. It is a little like putting the ring on the bride's finger.

"The well-prepared father is worth his weight in Demerol!" one nurse has said. I agree. Nothing can better relieve the mother's fear and pain in childbirth than a nurturing, well-informed birth partner.

Four essentials will enable the father to give effective labor support and enhance his own experience of the birth:

◆ *Learning about the laboring mind response.* Though the father should learn a little about the anatomy and physiology of labor, it is far more important for him to have some insight into the laboring mother's changing behavior and altered state of mind (see chapter 2).

◆ *Being nurturing.* The most valuable aid to the laboring mother is her birth partner's ability to give emotional and physical support (hugging, caressing her, and so on).

◆ *Learning about relaxation and guided imagery.*

◆ *Learning other ways of making the mother comfortable,* such as giving her a back massage, wiping her brow with compresses, and helping her change position.

Choosing Your Baby's Health Care Provider

The health care provider who attends your birth will do a newborn exam. However, it's best to choose your baby's health care provider for the weeks and months following birth during your pregnancy.

You may want to choose a pediatrician or family practitioner, or you may choose a well-baby clinic for general health care and a pediatrician for backup should consultation with a specialist be necessary.

When selecting your baby's health care provider:

◆ Choose one who fully supports breastfeeding, if this is how you plan to feed your baby. You might ask what percentage of the provider's clients breastfeed.

◆ Look for someone who answers your questions to your satisfaction.

◆ Look for someone who shares your philosophy regarding circumcision, immunizations, and whatever other aspects of baby care are important to you. (For more information on these subjects, see the Resources section of this book.)

Other points to consider are whether or not the health care provider charges for phone consultations, accepts insurance reimbursements (and, if so, whether or not the health care provider charges for filling out insurance forms), and, of course, whether he gets along well with you. As when selecting the health care provider who will attend your birth, you and your mate should choose your baby's health care provider together.

Who Else Will Attend the Birth?

A few expectant parents elect to give birth without anyone else, even a health care provider, present. Others prefer to have only their health care provider present. Still others want family, friends, and additional support persons to share the event.

If you choose to share your birth experience with others, be sure everyone who attends is fully supportive of your chosen method of childbirth. Being surrounded by supportive loved ones can empower a mother and make her feel secure. On the other hand, the stress and tension of having people present who think your birth method—for example, home birth—is tantamount to giving birth on a cliff's edge can cause you to have a longer, more difficult labor.

FAMILY AND FRIENDS AT BIRTH

An increasing number of expectant parents invite family and friends to share their birth. The presence of family and friends helps some mothers relax and feel more comfortable and supported during labor. The mother is able to experience the highs and lows of labor with familiar faces.

"I had everyone under the sun at my birth because it was something I wanted to share with a lot of people," recalls Kathy. "My mother-in-law came to take care of my other child, Mandy. I wanted to give her the gift of watching her grandchild being born. I wanted my sister and sisters-in-law there so they could see exactly what childbirth was like. I also invited my brother-in-law, a friend who was training to be a midwife, and the two midwives who were my primary birth attendants, as well as an extra one who was just there to give support and observe."

For many laboring women, family and friends at birth lessens fear. Continuous emotional support from loved ones is almost always associated with a more comfortable labor. In addition, being surrounded by familiar faces assists many women to better surrender to labor.

Needless to say, the mother should have the final choice about with whom she wants to share her birth. This is a basic human right, but, unfortunately, not a right protected by law. Many hospitals restrict the number of people the mother can have with her during labor. In the past some hospitals didn't even allow the father to attend unless he had taken special childbirth classes. Yet most hospitals that deny the laboring woman the guests of her choice have no trouble accommodating medical and nursing students.

Most childbearing centers place no restrictions on whom the mother invites to share her birth. And, of course, she can invite whomever she wants into her home. Hospitals, however, vary in their policies about the presence of others during labor. Some permit only one person to remain. A few place no restrictions on guests.

Be sure to select a birth place that honors the mother's right to have the guests of her choice, if you are planning a birth with others present.

Plan and discuss what role each person attending your birth will assume. Guests can help out in a wide variety of ways: taking photographs, replenishing warm compresses, giving emotional support, preparing a meal, and celebrating the event. Make sure your guests are aware that they will be expected to help.

CHILDREN ATTENDING BIRTH

I have visited hospitals that advertise themselves as offering "family-centered maternity care" yet don't even allow children to be present during the first hours after the baby is born, let alone during labor! Children are part of the family. There is no excuse for a policy that prevents children from participating in their own brother's or sister's arrival in the world.

In fact, sibling involvement at birth or during the immediate postpartum period may enhance their acceptance of the newcomer and decrease trauma.

Whether or not the family opts to have the children at the actual birth, they should certainly be included immediately afterward. They should be allowed to hold and touch the baby—not simply view the baby, like a fish in a tank, through the glass window of a nursery. In a good birth setting there are no restrictions about family participation.

"My daughter, four years old, sat next to me and held my hand during my labor," recalls one new mother. "At the last minute, she asked if she could let go and watch the baby being born and help Daddy and the midwife catch the baby."

Though always a miracle, birth seen through a child's eyes is especially magical. From tiny beginnings an unknown being grows in the mother's belly. During labor the baby leaves its snug and secure home to make a far more fabulous journey than could be made on the wings of a stork. One physician who attends both home and hospital births said that births with children present were the most unforgettable of all. Many childbirth professionals who have witnessed sibling-attended births agree.

When a child becomes a sibling, life changes dramatically and irreversibly. The child must make tremendous adjustments. He or she will no longer have the exclusive attention of mother and father but must learn to share their love. Involving children through pregnancy, birth, and the immediate postpartum period can ease this transition.

During birth children can help out in a variety of ways, depending on their age. A child can fan the mother, hold her hand, give her ice chips, serve her food and liquids, replenish hot or cold compresses, and assist the father by doing other odd jobs as the need arises.

Your child should be able to come and go so that he or she does not have to be cooped up in one room for an extended period. A childbearing center or hospital with a separate play area for children is ideal, but a hospital lobby, cafeteria, and the street outside can provide needed distractions.

Another adult or older child should be present to care for children under four. Some children may want or need to leave the birth place from time to time, especially if your labor is long.

Many parents are surprised to discover how children take the childbearing drama in stride. When well prepared, most children take labor and birth for granted. On the other hand, little is as wondrous as the face of a brother or sister during the unfolding miracle. Birth through a child's eyes is like Christmas morning. Her eyes widen. A radiant smile breaks across her face. The room pulses with energy. There is no question a miracle has occurred.

Preparing Children for Birth

You should prepare children for birth in advance. We involved both of our sons early in our preparation for our third child. We began by asking them how they felt about having a new brother or sister. Once the baby was conceived, they were actively included through the pregnancy and postpartum weeks.

When we were preparing for our son Jonathan's birth, our three-year-old son, Paul, said, "I want to be a mommy too!" I'll always remember how he cried when we told him boys couldn't be mommies. His brother Carl, six years old, had a different reaction.

"When my brother, Paul, and I found out we were going to have a new baby in the family, we all started preparing," recalls Carl. "We read books about how babies grow inside their mothers and how babies are born. Mom and Dad showed us pictures of babies being born so we would know what to expect.

"We went shopping for baby clothes and other things. Sometimes that was fun. And sometimes it was real boring.

"Paul and I went to the midwife's appointments with Mom and Dad. We heard the baby's heart beat!

"The night before the baby was born, I visited my grandma's while Paul stayed home. Before I went to bed, I reminded Grandma to wake me up if my mom went into labor. When she woke me up in the middle of the night, I didn't know where I was at first.

"'What's going on?' I asked. She told me. We rushed to our apartment. Grandma drove fast. She went through a red light.

"When I got there, the baby was already born! I was sad because I wanted to see the birth. But I was also real excited. I woke up Paul. We both saw Daddy cut the umbilical cord.

"And now we are getting ready to have another baby!"

Fortunately, three years later, when Carl was nine, he made up for not being present at the birth. He witnessed and helped with the birth of his youngest brother, Eric. The following is excerpted from an article he wrote at the time, an account that can teach every parent and child about preparing children for the newcomer.

Today we brought our new baby mountain hiking for the first time. He just turned three weeks old. My mom carried Eric up the mountain in a cloth baby carrier. My dad carried the backpack and the water container.

On the way to the top we met some people climbing over the steep rocks on their way down the trail. They stopped and talked and asked how old he was. They were amazed to see a new baby on the trail! I guess there usually aren't too many newborns on mountain trails.

When we got to the top of the mountain, my mom breastfed the baby. He was real hungry after the long climb.

We could see a long way away from the mountain top. But Eric didn't seem to notice the great view. He was too busy eating.

I'll always remember when I saw him born three weeks ago.

Before Mom was pregnant, she asked me if I wanted a new baby. I told her I really did. I really wanted a brother. But a sister was okay too.

When Mom got pregnant, we spent a long time getting ready to have the baby. We went through clothes. And every night we read a book about having a baby. I looked at pictures showing babies in their mothers and babies being born.

I learned a lot of things.

I learned how brothers and sisters can help during labor. They can bring cool drinks to their mom. They can hold their mom's hand. And they can bring stuff that the midwife needs.

I learned about labor and how babies get born. It's real hard work. I learned what the placenta looks like. I learned how the cord looks. I was surprised it was white. I also learned there might be a lot of blood after the placenta comes out. And I remembered that mothers might make strange noises when a baby is born.

My brothers and I went to each appointment at the doctor's with my mom and dad. He asked how Mom felt and we listened to the baby's heart. We were going to a doctor just in case we needed him. But my dad was going to catch the baby.

We also went to a midwife. She lived in a house in the woods. She was going to help us in the hospital if we needed her.

On Friday when Eric was born, I woke up about 4 o'clock

in the morning. I heard my Mom and Dad talking about the baby. My Mom was making strange sounds.

I knew that we might have the baby soon! Very quietly I got up and turned on the light. Nobody knew I was up. I woke my brother Paul and told him we might have the baby! I got dressed.

Then I got back in bed and waited quietly.

A few minutes later my dad came into my room. "Do you want to go to the birth?" he asked.

I sat up in bed and said, "I really want to go!"

He was amazed to see I was awake and dressed!

He told me to wake my youngest brother, Jonathan. Paul was already up and getting dressed.

In a little while, my brothers and I went to the car and waited for my mom and dad to come.

On the way to the hospital my mom was making some more strange noises. Paul and I were a little scared that we might have the baby in the car!

We got to the hospital about 5:00 A.M. Our midwife was waiting for us in the parking lot.

A few minutes later we were in the birth room. My mom was pushing the baby out. My dad said, "Come look at the baby's head coming out!"

I was real excited to see the baby's head come out!

My Dad was helping with his hands on the baby's head. Then the midwife started helping.

I didn't like the way the baby's head looked as it was coming out. It looked like it had a lot of soap on it. I turned away for a few seconds. My dad told me that the greasy stuff on the baby's head and body is called vernix and is like hand cream. It protects the baby's skin while he is in the uterus.

When I turned back, the whole baby was out!

Right after the baby was born, the midwife put blankets on him. Nobody else saw whether it was a boy or girl, not even the midwife. But I knew. I had seen that it was a boy.

After my mom was holding the baby for a couple of minutes, I told her it was a boy.

My dad cut the cord while my mom breastfed the baby.

In a little while the placenta came out. I didn't like the way it looked at all! It looked like a huge piece of liver on one side and a rock on the other side.

A few minutes later my grandma came into the birth room. She had driven a long way to get there. But she missed the birth.

Then the doctor came. He was a little disappointed he missed the birth too!

I'm glad I saw Eric being born! It is wonderful to see your own baby brother born!

My brothers and I sat all together on a big chair in the birth room, feeling real excited watching my mom feed Eric. Then after about an hour Jonathan said, "Why are we staying here so long?" He wanted to play cars with Eric at home.

We stayed a little while longer because my mom wanted to take a shower.

And about 7:00 A.M. we went home.

I helped my dad cook breakfast.

The day Mom had the baby, she was in the living room breastfeeding for most of the day. Grandma and Dad helped around the house.

But the next day she was like she always was before the birth. She wanted to mow the lawn. But it was raining outside. So she didn't mow the lawn until the day after. When the midwife came to our home, she was very surprised to see my mom mowing the lawn.

My dad says that most women rest for days after having a baby. But my Mom never does. She is always up and doing things a few hours after having a baby.

I like to hold the baby. He is so tiny. He holds my finger with his hand. He likes it when I hold him.

I don't like to hear him crying because I want him to be

happy. He stops crying when I pick him up, unless he's real
hungry. When the baby wakes up, I get him from his
cradle and bring him to my mom so she can breastfeed
him.

I'm very happy about having a new brother!

The following steps—all implicit in Carl's article—will help
prepare your child for birth and the transition to becoming a
brother or sister.

- ◆ *Choose a health care provider and, if you are planning an out-
  of-home birth, a childbearing center or hospital supportive of
  children at birth.* Remember, even some hospitals that call
  themselves "family-centered" do not allow children at
  birth. Phone the health care provider or childbearing
  center and ask how many parents elect to have their
  children present during labor. You might want to ask what
  suggestions they have for preparing a child for birth.
  Should the reaction be less than positive, consider another
  health care provider and birth place.

Some parents choose their birth place for the sake of being
able to have their children present. Helen's story is an example.
The mother of four boys, Helen was pregnant with her fifth child,
whom she hoped would be a girl! The first four births took place in
a local hospital. But this time Helen wanted a family birth with her
four sons present. Since no hospital in her area allowed children to
attend births, she planned a home birth. When it was time to push
her baby out into the world, Helen lay back on her bed propped up
on pillows like a queen. The father sat next to her and rubbed her
back. The four boys at the end of the bed were breathless,
anticipating the birth of their sister. As the baby's head started to
show, the boys were wide-eyed with awe. The rest of the body
slipped out. There was a moment of silence. Then four grins broke
across the boys' faces and soft chuckling filled the air. The mother
reached down to take her child. "Oh, my God!" she hollered as she
took her fifth son lovingly to her breast.

- ◆ *Educate your children about birth.* "How is the baby going to
  pop out?" our three-year-old son Paul asked. He could
  understand how the child grew in the mother's uterus, but

how it would get out was another matter. Paul is not alone. Even though they are acquainted with the anatomy of birth, most mothers and fathers wonder the same thing! Tell your child what to expect during labor and birth. Be sure to include the delivery of the placenta. Let your child know that there will be a considerable amount of blood so it will not be a shock.

◆ *Be sure to mention how some mothers moan, sigh, and even scream at times.* If you are vocal in your labor, this will come as less of a surprise.

◆ *Give your child a realistic idea of how newborns look and behave.* Explain that for the first weeks of life newborns don't look much like the babies in baby food advertisements. Furthermore, children should that know newborns are not very exciting playmates. Many children are disappointed to find that the newborn is interested only in eating and sleeping. You can nevertheless involve your children in the infant's life. Depending on your child's age, you can acquaint him or her with ways to help out, from changing diapers to sharing a bath with the newborn.

◆ *Include your children at prenatal appointments.* As pregnancy unfolds, your child should meet your health care provider. At prenatal appointments the sibling-to-be can listen to the fetal heartbeat through a fetoscope (special stethoscope for hearing heart tones). He or she can also ask questions. Some midwives and physicians have birth picture books the child can look at to learn about the birth process while waiting for the exam. If you are planning to give birth in a childbearing center or hospital, take your child to visit the birth place. Seeing where Mom and Dad will be acquaints the child with what to expect.

◆ *Shop for the layette with your children.* Shopping for the baby clothes, toys, and furniture can also help a child of any age confront his or her feelings and adjust to the fact that there will be a new family member. Psychiatrist Martin Greenberg, whose pioneer research in the area of paternal-infant bonding is well known, told me that while shopping for the layette with his wife he was utterly surprised to see how tiny newborn clothing was. It was a striking revelation about how vulnerable and dependent his new child would be. If a physician who is intimately acquainted with newborns finds the size of infant clothing a surprise, imagine how a child feels! Shopping for the layette is a good opportunity to explain that the newcomer will be wholly dependent on Mother for a while and, therefore, will need the lion's share of attention. This is an important issue to confront before your baby is born, and conveying it to your other children will make your life more comfortable and serene afterward.

Some childbirth educators hold sibling preparation classes. These classes vary greatly. Some are designed to prepare a child for becoming a brother or sister but not necessarily to attend the birth. Others prepare the child to participate in the birth. You may want to consider bringing your child to one of your own childbirth classes. This can be helpful especially if a birth film is shown. A few educational films show children at birth. If you would like to view such a film, call local childbirth educators and ask if they have a film depicting children at birth that you can make arrangements to see.

After the twentieth week of pregnancy, with a hand on the mother's abdomen, your child can feel the baby move. For siblings this can be a turning point, marking the time when the pregnancy stops being a big belly and becomes a little brother or sister.

After the Birth

A colleague once told me that the tales of women who give birth only to return to work immediately afterward are fictional. Women can't really do that, she claimed. But she was wrong: that's just what Jan did after the births of all our children. When our third child, Jonathan, was born, we were house hunting a day later, four hours from our home. Within an hour after the birth of our fourth child, Eric, Jan was up cooking a meal, while I, on the other hand, was so exhausted I could barely walk! Yes, we arranged for help around the home—as all parents *should*—but Jan hardly required it!

As long as there are no medical complications, you can be up and about as soon as you want after birth. The father can help you the first time you get out of bed in case you feel dizzy, lightheaded, weak in the knees, or faint. You will require plenty of rest during the postpartum period—even if you are one of those unusual women, like Jan, who insist on being active immediately after giving birth. (Jan finally did sit down at the insistence of our midwife!) Limit your activities to taking care of yourself and your baby for the first week or so after birth.

Plan to have help around the home. The life-altering era after the birth of your baby is no time to try to be self-sufficient. It is quite appropriate to depend on your family and perhaps friends for a few days or longer.

The father can take charge of all household responsibilities, but he should not try to do all the work himself. I suggest that he delegate most of the work to family members, friends, or perhaps hired help. He too needs time to adjust to his new baby, and he will also probably need rest.

I'll never forget how much it meant to us when my own mother helped Jan and me after our second son, Paul, was born. She stayed with us for a few days, cooked, cleaned, shopped, and even took little trips with Carl, who was then two years old.

"My mother and my husband's mother came to our home from time to time to clean up and cook, and friends brought food," recalls Ann of the days after her baby was born. "This gave me time to rest and be with my daughter, who wanted to nurse constantly."

One couple, Jean and Tony, belong to a church that sends meals to parents' homes for two weeks after birth—a great gift for the new family.

You may want to let relatives know you would appreciate a home-cooked meal or other help for a baby gift.

Family members and friends should focus on the new parents' needs—especially by helping out at home rather than assuming baby care responsibilities. Of course, grandparents will find it irresistible to spend some time cuddling the baby. And you can hardly expect anyone to do the hard work without being allowed to enjoy the best part! But you as the parent should take on the role of baby care and learn to trust your own ability—even though you may feel awkward or want to rely on others at first.

Be sure the persons who are helping out are supportive of your chosen method of childbirth, breastfeeding, and whatever aspects of parenting are important to you. It does little good to have relatives around who are constantly criticizing your parenting style.

Try to limit visitors. Even helpful visitors can be exhausting for the new family. As in most everything in childbearing, let your feelings—physical and emotional—be your guide.

PATERNITY LEAVE

Martin, a new father, remained home for a week after the birth of his child. His paternity leave was unpaid. "I can't imagine how I would have done it if I hadn't had him home!" exclaims his wife, Cheri. "I have one flat and one inverted nipple and had some problems breastfeeding. We didn't know anyone who had breastfed, but Martin was very supportive. In the middle of the night when I was exhausted and had absolutely no patience, he was able to be there for me when I needed him."

I strongly urge every new father—regardless of where the birth takes place—to take a week to be with his unfolding family and help out around the home. Though most men won't be paid for the time off, they'll find that the benefits of taking paternity leave outweigh the financial loss. The father will find it easier to adjust to his new fathering role if he is with his family for a few days without interruption. He can help out with the cooking, cleaning, laundry, and other chores, and give the mother much-needed emotional support. As a final benefit he can rest.

"I stayed in bed for most of the first week after birth, getting up just to shower and change diapers," Maryann recalls. "Mark did the cooking and cleaning. When I wanted to take a nap, he'd take the baby and sleep with her on the couch until she wanted to nurse."

In my opinion, the father should take paternity leave whether or not the parents have others to help out around the home or plan to hire professional help. *Nothing substitutes for the father's presence.* Though there may be others to meet the mother's practical needs, the father is still needed to cope with the emotional adjustments and realities of shared parenthood.

THE POSTPARTUM COMPANION

In many areas, professional postpartum companions are available to new families. Such people now often replace or assist the mother or grandmother who traditionally helped the new mother through the first few days after the birth a few generations ago.

Postpartum companions do a wide variety of jobs from house cleaning and cooking to giving breastfeeding help. Many take vital signs (temperature, pulse, and respiration), examine the mother to ensure that she is recovering properly, and answer basic health questions.

The services of these professionals are becoming increasingly widespread as more and more families opt for early discharge from hospitals or plan to give birth at home or in childbearing centers.

GETTING THE INFORMATION YOU NEED

Phone numbers of persons who can answer questions about breastfeeding and give you other health information should be available at your fingertips after the baby is born.

For a breastfeeding specialist, get the telephone number of a lactation consultant, a local nursing mothers' information service, or a La Leche League group. Lactation consultants are highly trained professionals who charge for their services. Local nursing mothers' information services are available through many childbirth education organizations. A nursing counselor may be able to talk with you on the phone and perhaps even visit your home at no charge, and local maternity units are also willing to answer questions over the phone.

Any local childbirth educator should be able to give you telephone numbers. Most are willing to answer questions about baby care and maternal health issues. If you have taken childbirth classes, have your childbirth educator's telephone number handy. La Leche League International (LLLI) is a worldwide organization that provides information in most cities in the United States. If you can't find a local branch of LLLI listed in your phone directory, call the national office for a referral. (See Resources at the end of this book.)

Before you complete your birth options plan, you should be thoroughly familiar with all your birth choices and all the common obstetrical routines and procedures. These are discussed in detail in the next chapter.

By planning your birth carefully, you are doing more than just increasing your chances of a safe, rewarding birth experience for you and your family. You are acquainting health professionals with contemporary expectant parents' needs, and will thereby help to shape childbirth for the future.

Obstetric Routines and Procedures

In the United States and Canada a wide variety of obstetrical routines and procedures are common both during normal birth and birth with medical complications. According to pediatrician and epidemiologist Marsden G. Wagner of the World Health Organization, "Obstetrical intervention rates in the United States far exceed those of any country in Europe. Indeed, the cesarean section rate in the United States ranges from nearly double to over triple that of the European countries.... Countries with some of the lowest perinatal mortality rates in the world have cesarean section rates of less than 10 percent."[1] The Dutch, for example, use such obstetrical procedures as episiotomy rarely and only if there are genuine medical complications. For this reason Dutch parents have less trouble educating themselves about maternity care options and drawing up a birth options plan.

Medical routines are so common in the United States and Canada, however, that all American and Canadian parents must take it upon themselves to learn the advantages and disadvantages of all common procedures in their area if they want to plan a safe, rewarding birth experience for themselves and their family.

Make a conscious, well-informed choice about *all* procedures and routines common in your area. Include each in your birth options plan as necessary. Don't make your plan longer than it need be, by including irrelevant information. For example, if you've selected an obstetrician who encourages women to adopt the position of their choice during labor and birth, it is hardly necessary to include this in your birth options plan.

For the safest, most rewarding birth experience, avoid all unnecessary obstetrical intervention. Unnecessary interventions may include shaving of the perineal area, administration of an enema, intravenous feeding, electronic fetal monitoring, artificial rupture of the membranes, oxytocic drugs (Pitocin) to augment labor, and episiotomy. We will discuss each of these in detail.

In rare circumstances each of these procedures has its place. In some hospitals, however, obstetrical procedures designed for high risk-labor have become routine.

If it works, don't fix it. Otherwise it might really break down.

Labor is the only natural process medical professionals have turned into a clinical procedure. Behind the scenes of many conventional hospitals is the view that birth is a medical crisis where technical help is needed every step of the way. Contrast this to the following view: Dr. G. J. Kloosterman, professor of obstetrics at the University of Amsterdam, asserts "childbirth in itself is a natural phenomenon and in the large majority of cases needs no interference whatsoever—only close observation, moral support, and protection against human meddling."[2]

In some hospitals one or more of the procedures described below may be routine to the point of being almost mandatory. If you elect to avoid a particular procedure, from use of intravenous feeding to electronic fetal monitoring (and the choice is *always* yours), a physician or nurse may ask you to sign a form stating that you are refusing the procedure "against medical advice." However, if you create a birth options plan and discuss the details thoroughly with your health care providers, the form shouldn't be necessary.

It bears repeating: *Routine medical intervention can actually cause the very problems they were designed to prevent.*

First we will discuss procedures done during labor, then we'll cover those relating to the immediate postpartum period.

First-Stage Labor

PERINEAL PREPPING

Avoid having the perineal area shaved. Shaving or clipping the hair around the birth outlet, sometimes called "prepping," is still routine in a few hospitals; though, for the most part, this curious custom is falling out of favor. In the past prepping was thought to reduce the chance of infection. But in fact, research reveals that prepping may even increase the possibility of infection![3] Also, shaving the pubic hair causes the new mother discomfort while the hair grows back. With a new baby on her hands, the last thing she needs is perineal itch.

ENEMA

Avoid an enema unless you really want to clear the bowels or to stimulate an overdue labor. In some hospitals the laboring woman is given an enema shortly after admission, though like prepping, this procedure is becoming less common. The enema's purpose is to clear the bowels prior to birth. However, prelabor diarrhea usually does this effectively. It is common for a little stool to be released during birth. This is simply wiped away and scarcely noticed.

Some mothers find the enema very uncomfortable, particularly during late labor. For those who feel they'd like one, a self-administered enema is usually preferable to one administered by a stranger. Do the enema during early labor when it is less uncomfortable.

INTRAVENOUS FEEDING

Avoid intravenous feeding (IV) unless you have a medical complication requiring you to receive medication by this route. The IV replaces normal fluid and food consumption in a few hospital labor and delivery units. Those who favor IVs for laboring women claim that the IV will make it easier to administer medication or an immediate blood transfusion should such be required. This is like advocating routine intravenous feeding in automobiles—just in case an accident occurs requiring a blood transfusion.

Few will disagree that intravenous feeding has its place in the treatment of the ill. If the mother is unable to take liquids by mouth for some reason, the IV may be justified during labor to prevent dehydration or hypoglycemia (low blood sugar). But most contemporary childbirth educators agree that IVs have no place in normal labor. The IV makes most laboring mothers feel like invalids, impairs mobility, and, by so doing, impairs labor.

Alternatives to Intravenous Feeding

Drink and eat to satisfy your body's needs and maintain your health. Strange as it may seem, a few conventional hospitals withhold food and liquids by mouth from laboring mothers. This policy was instituted when a high percentage of mothers gave birth under general anesthesia, with the risk of vomiting while unconscious and asphyxiating on the stomach's contents. However, few receive general anesthesia today, and those who do are intubated, to prevent them from aspirating regurgitated stomach contents. Yet the policy remains, like stale food after a party.

Nurses frequently offer ice chips to laboring women to quench thirst. Ice chips may be welcome, especially if the mother is sweaty. But they aren't much of a substitute for nourishing liquids and food! Labor is hard work. You deserve a decent meal.

You will especially need nourishment if your labor is long. The IV supplies energy but is no substitute for eating and drinking normally. Avoiding food can cause you to have a longer labor and become exhausted.

Digestion may slow during labor but doesn't stop altogether. Most women enjoy hot tea with honey or fruit juice. It is best to eat lightly—gelatin, hot soup, toast with jam, and so forth.

As in most everything in childbirth, let your body be your guide about when and how much to eat and drink.

ARTIFICIAL RUPTURE OF THE MEMBRANES

Avoid artificial rupture of the membranes (ROM) unless your condition warrants it, as in the case of a prolonged labor that is not progressing after *all* the suggestions listed in the section on alternatives to Pitocin (pp. 95–96) have been tried. The intentional rupturing of the membranes, also called amniotomy, is a common procedure in many hospitals. A nurse or the primary health care provider ruptures the membranes (amniotic sac) during early or middle labor, using either a finger or, more commonly, a long plastic hook shaped somewhat like a crochet needle. This usually painless procedure is done to speed up labor or to allow an electrode for an internal fetal monitor to be attached. Numerous researchers have pointed out several disadvantages and risks to both mother and baby associated with artificial ROM.[4] The amniotic fluid provides a sterile environment and cushions the baby during uterine contractions so that pressure is evenly distributed. In most hospitals, once the membranes are ruptured, the clock is set in motion. The mother is generally expected to give birth within twenty-four hours (to reduce the chance of infection) and may be given Pitocin to augment labor. In addition, after ROM, compression of the umbilical cord and perhaps a fall in uterine blood flow may contribute to fetal distress, which can and often does lead to a cesarean.

The advantages of amniotomy are that

◆ It sometimes shortens labor
◆ It sometimes initiates an overdue labor

The disadvantages of amniotomy are that

◆ It may cause more painful contractions
◆ There is an increased risk of infection
◆ There is potential damage to the soft bones of the baby's skull
◆ It may cause oxygen deprivation by compressing the umbilical cord[5]
◆ It increases the likelihood of a cesarean section

Alternatives to Amniotomy

Though amniotomy can sometimes shorten labor by about an hour, the benefits of this procedure are at best inconsistent and unpredictable.[6] Dr. Roberto Caldeyro-Barcia, former president of the International Federation of Gynecologists and Obstetricians and director of the Latin American Center of Perinatology and Human Development for the World Health Organization, points out that "Acceleration of labor is not necessarily beneficial for the fetus and newborn and it may be associated with poor outcome for the offspring."[7]

Other more natural ways of shortening labor include a vertical rather than horizontal position for the laboring women, physical and emotional support from a birth partner, and a peaceful setting where the laboring woman's emotional as well as physical needs are met. Occasionally, however, ROM is beneficial when other methods of accelerating labor won't help, but *other methods should be tried first*. During late labor some women find rupturing the membranes a relief. But whether or not the membranes are ruptured should always be your decision.

ELECTRONIC FETAL MONITORING

Make a conscious decision regarding electronic fetal monitoring (EFM) based on your own research and your intuitive reaction. Thousands of articles pro and con have been published about EFM. I recommend reading a few of the most recent ones both for and against the procedure, then making a decision based on your own comfort, unless you have a medical complication that may warrant EFM.

The electronic fetal monitor (EFM) is a machine that records both fetal heart rate (FHR) and the intensity of uterine contractions on a continuous sheet of graph paper. There are two basic types of monitoring, external and internal.

External monitoring: Two straps, attached to a nearby machine, are placed around the mother's abdomen. On one, an ultrasound transducer picks up the FHR. On the other, a pressure-sensitive device detects the intensity of uterine contractions.

Internal monitoring: The health care provider passes a wire through the vagina and cervix and attaches it to the baby's scalp to pick up the FHR. Then he or she inserts a fluid-filled, pressure-sensitive catheter into the uterus to determine the intensity of contractions. (Often the FHR is monitored internally while contractions are monitored externally.) Internal monitoring is more accurate but also more complicated and invasive.

Most physicians believe EFM has a valid place in the obstetrical care of high-risk labors. This is why the monitor was originally introduced. However, like mushrooms after an autumn rain, electronic fetal monitors have suddenly appeared in hospitals across the nation and have become routine in normal labor. According to a report issued by the National Institutes of Health, "Present evidence does not show benefit of electronic fetal monitoring to low-risk patients."[8]

In fact, EFM can *disrupt* normal labor. This is, no doubt, the reason the cesarean rate for impaired labor has proved to be as much as double among electronically monitored mothers. In an often-quoted study Dr. Albert Haverkamp and three other physicians divided 483 mothers of similar risk status into two groups. One group had EFM. In the other, a nurse listened to the FHR through a fetoscope. Among the monitored mothers, the cesarean rate was 2.5 times higher, with no difference in the baby's wellbeing. Apgar scores (a measure of the newborn's color, heart rate, respiration, reflex response and muscle tone)* taken at one minute after birth were similar in both groups. However, the Apgar scores five minutes after birth were superior in the group without EFM.[9] There was also a dramatic increase in postpartum infection among the EFM mothers.

The results surprised Dr. Haverkamp. He discovered that contrary to the beliefs of many conscientious obstetricians, EFM is "not associated with an improvement in perinatal outcome." He admits, "We expected that the electronically monitored infants would be in better condition than those who were merely auscultated [monitored by fetoscope] since signs of distress could be acted upon more speedily."[10]

Drs. Howard L. Minkoff and Richard H. Schwartz have called attention to "the stress a monitored patient may experience because of the use of noisy, incomprehensible machines."[11] Stress is associated with the release of catecholamines (stress hormones, such as adrenaline), and their release may narrow the blood vessels and reduce the fetal heart rate. Several other physicians have clearly demonstrated a correlation between use of EFM and increased cesareans. A study published in the *New England Journal of Medicine* showed that there was no benefit to the use of EFM during premature labors. In fact, a higher cerebral palsy rate was observed with the continuously monitored group.[12]

EFM shows that obstetrics is often less a science than a belief system with people holding opposing views. People who believe in routine EFM defend the machine with near-religious fervor, while others think it has no place in normal birth.

Despite the studies showing the potential hazards of monitoring, EFM is becoming more, rather than less, popular. One reason

*The Apgar score is a number from 0 to 10 determined at one and five minutes after birth. Each of the five physical signs—color, heart rate, respiration, reflex response, and muscle tone is given a score of 0, 1, or 2. The total of the five scores is the Apgar score. The highest posible Apgar score is 10.

is that the machine saves nursing time. Intermittent monitoring by less invasive means requires hands-on care by a skilled nurse.

The advantage of electronic fetal monitoring is that

◆ It reveals fetal distress.

The disadvantages of electronic fetal monitoring are that

◆ Mothers tend to be in a supine position when having EFM, leading to fetal oxygen deprivation.
◆ It inhibits mobility during labor, which interferes with normal labor and may lead to fetal distress.
◆ It inhibits the ability of the birth partner to provide the close, caressing labor support the mother usually requires.
◆ Internal monitoring requires rupture of the membranes, which carries its own risks of infection.
◆ It inhibits the mother's spontaneous reaction to labor.
◆ Monitors frequently malfunction, giving erroneous information.
◆ Less common mishaps, including fetal scalp abscess and accidents to the baby from internal monitor electrodes, do sometimes occur.

Alternatives to Electronic Fetal Monitoring

There are two other methods of monitoring the fetal heart: the practitioner *auscultates* (listens to) the baby's heart rate with a special stethoscope called a fetoscope. Or the heart tones can be heard with a Doppler, a hand-held ultrasound device that amplifies the fetal heart sounds.

Labor Positions

You will almost invariably adopt the best labor position by following your own intuition. Be sure to adopt the position of your choice unless you suffer a medical emergency requiring bed rest. Find the position that works best for you during first-stage labor as the cervix dilates and during second-stage labor as your baby is born.

FIRST STAGE

Generally speaking, upright positions such as standing, sitting, and walking are best for first-stage labor. Some women feel comfortable kneeling on all fours. Health professionals in most contemporary birth settings encourage you to labor in a semireclining position when electronic fetal monitoring is engaged.

The advantages of vertical positions during first-stage labor are that

+ They decrease discomfort.
+ They increase the speed of labor.
+ They may decrease the incidence of fetal distress.[13]

The disadvantages of the back-lying position during first-stage labor are that

+ It contributes to a longer, more difficult labor.
+ It can cause maternal hypotension (low blood pressure) by putting pressure on the inferior vena cava (major artery), thereby reducing the oxygen reaching the baby and causing fetal distress.

SECOND STAGE

As the story goes, a large truck tried to pass under a bridge that was too low. The truck got jammed in the center with its roof wedged under the bottom of the bridge. The truck driver couldn't figure out what to do, nor could the tow truck driver or the police. While they were standing around talking about removing the truck's roof, or even temporarily relocating the girders, a little boy came to watch. The boy said, "Why don't you let the air out of the tires?"

I've seen quite a few American maternity units that could benefit from such common sense. I've often observed nurses tell a mother to push in a back-lying position when it was obvious she was making no progress. This situation is so nonsensical it would be hard to believe if it didn't occur so often! Stirrups were invented by the ancient Scythians for riding horses, not for having babies. Today stirrups may be useful for certain gynecological procedures or for the repair of lacerations and use of forceps when truly necessary, but avoid them for normal birth.

Dr. Roberto Caldeyro-Barcia has called the lithotomy position (flat on the back with feet in stirrups) the worst position for labor except for being hung by the feet.[14]

This position was popularized for the convenience of the health care provider, not for the mother's comfort. In many hospitals the mother now gives birth in a semireclining position instead.

In striking contrast to Western custom, in the majority of non-European, non-U.S. countries, women give birth in some form of upright position—sitting, squatting, on hands and knees, or standing with support.[15]

The advantages of birth in an upright position are that

◆ The birth canal is slightly shortened as the pelvic outlet is expanded—by an average of 28 percent in the squatting, as compared to the supine, position.

◆ Gravity is on the squatting woman's side; squatting can shorten an otherwise long bearing-down stage and is especially helpful if the baby is in a posterior position.

The disadvantages of back-lying or using stirrups during birth are that

◆ Pushing is more difficult (as the mother pushes against gravity).

◆ Birth is more difficult.

◆ Pain is increased.

◆ The risk of perineal lacerations is increased.

◆ Blood flow to the uterus is decreased (with its associated potential for fetal oxygen deprivation), resulting from constriction of the mothers' blood vessels.[16]

◆ The risk of having an episiotomy is greater.

◆ The risk of forceps delivery is greater.

Pain-Relief Medication

Use nonpharmacological pain relief methods before resorting to pain relief medication. All obstetrical analgesia and anesthesia affect uterine contractions and can impair labor. No medication has proven entirely safe for the baby. In addition, the use of pain medication frequently breeds more intervention. For example, drugs can slow labor down, causing the health care provider to initiate hormonal augmentation, which may in turn precipitate the need for a cesarean. For example, I recently conducted a workshop for the childbirth professionals in a Southern hospital where 90 percent of mothers have epidural anesthesia, which numbs the body from the chest down. Expectant mothers were actually given classes to prepare for epidural anesthesia. The cesarean rate at that hospital is over 40 percent.

According to Dr. John B. Caire of Lake Charles Memorial Hospital in Lake Charles, Louisiana, the use of regional anesthesia (epidural, spinal, caudal, saddleblock, and so forth) reduces labor's effectiveness, causes various degrees of fetal *anoxia* (inadequate oxygen supply), and hinders the bearing-down process.[17]

Women who plan their birth carefully and have good labor support in an emotionally positive environment use dramatically less pain relief medication than mothers who give birth in settings that are not conducive to a spontaneous reaction. The use of analgesia is very rare during home birth. And in most childbearing centers, pain medication is not even available. However, even in childbearing centers where medication is readily available, women rarely find the need to request it. In one survey of 4,500 women giving birth in a hospital-owned childbearing center, fewer than 4 percent requested analgesia.[18]

Two basic types of pain-relief medication are available: *analgesia* reduces pain, oftentimes used in conjunction with tranquilizers and sedatives, and *anesthesia* eliminates pain. We will discuss each separately.

ANALGESIA

A variety of narcotic analgesics are used to reduce pain in labor. Meperidine (Demerol) is the most widely used.

The advantages of narcotic analgesics include

◆ Reduced pain
◆ Promotion of sleep and relaxation, which can sometimes accelerate labor

The disadvantages of narcotic analgesics include

◆ Nausea
◆ Drowsiness
◆ Prolonged labor (sometimes)
◆ Reduced ability by the mother to participate in the childbearing experience
◆ Depression of the baby's central nervous system (most likely when the medication is given four hours or less before birth)

TRANQUILIZERS

Tranquilizers are used to reduce anxiety and increase the effects of narcotic analgesia so that less narcotic is necessary.

The advantages of tranquilizers are

◆ Reduced anxiety
◆ Reduced nausea and vomiting from analgesia
◆ Enhanced effects of narcotic analgesia

The disadvantages of tranquilizers are

For the mother:

◆ Nausea
◆ Drowsiness
◆ Confusion
◆ Prolonged labor
◆ Reduced blood pressure
◆ Urinary retention

- Dry mouth
- Pain at the injection site
- Reduced ability by the mother to participate in the childbearing experience

For the baby:

- An increased risk of hypothermia (low body temperature) and poor muscle tone, with a large dose
- An increased risk of too much bilirubin in the baby's system, leading to jaundice
- Enhanced negative effects of narcotic analgesia

SEDATIVES

Like tranquilizers, sedatives are another class of medication used to reduce anxiety and sometimes induce sleep. In addition, sedatives facilitate the use of such other procedures as forceps delivery.

The advantages of sedatives are

- Reduced anxiety
- Promotion of relaxation and sleep
- Altered pain perception

The disadvantages of sedatives are

- Dizziness
- Nausea
- Possible hypotension (low blood pressure)
- Reduced ability by the mother to participate in the childbearing experience
- Delayed responses in the baby
- Increased risk for the baby of respiratory problems

ALTERNATIVES TO PAIN-RELIEF MEDICATION, TRANQUILIZERS, AND SEDATIVES

What are the alternatives to all these medications? Continuous labor support; guided imagery; an emotionally positive birth setting; a psychologically compatible health care provider; use of comfort measures, including relaxation, breathing patterns, warm baths, and showers; massage; changing positions and walking as desired; and eating and drinking to satisfy the body's needs. If you use *all* of these, your chances of needing pain-relief medication, tranquilizers, or sedatives approach zero.

REGIONAL ANESTHESIA

Regional anesthesia blocks sensation in parts of your body while allowing you to remain conscious. Several types of regional anesthesia are used for labor. These include epidural block, paracervical block, pudendal block, and local anesthesia, among others. Local anesthesia is used prior to an episiotomy or to stitch tears after birth.

Epidural Anesthesia

Epidural anesthesia is the most frequently used anesthesia for labor in the United States and Canada. Effective within fifteen minutes, it numbs the body from chest to toes and renders the area temporarily immobile.

New forms of epidural anesthesia have been developed that use a small amount of an anesthetic agent, such as lidocaine, mixed with a small quantity of a narcotic analgesic such as morphine. The two act synergistically, that is, the total effect of the mixture is far greater than what you'd expect from adding together the separate effects. (In a synergistic relationship, the sum is greater than the added parts.) Anesthesiologists have some question whether to call this epidural anesthesia or analgesia. Its relative safety and the fact that mobility is usually possible with this new form of epidural anesthesia have made it extremely popular.

The anesthesiologist usually administers the epidural when the cervix is dilated four or five centimeters, sometimes earlier and sometimes later, depending on the situation. While the mother sits up or lies curled on her side, the anesthetic agent is injected into the spinal canal region, but the needle does not penetrate the dura (thick outer covering of the spinal cord.) A thin tube is left in the mother's back so that more anesthesia can be injected as needed.

The epidural anesthesia rate is rising dramatically, particularly with improvements rendering the procedure increasingly safe. Epidural anesthesia is effective and usually the anesthesia of choice for cesarean delivery.

The advantages of epidural anesthesia are

- Pain relief through first- and second-stage labor
- Ease of maintaining the anesthesia via the catheter
- Facilitated use of forceps

The disadvantages of epidural anesthesia are

For the mother:

- Possible lack of mobility throughout labor (depending on type used)
- Hypotension
- Increased need for Pitocin to induce or augment labor (see p. 95)
- Increased incidence of forceps delivery
- Increased risk of a more extensive episiotomy or lacerations
- Increased risk of cesarean surgery
- "Necessity" of electronic fetal monitoring

For the baby:

- Risk for the baby of bradycardia (low heart rate)
- Increased chance of fetal distress
- Possible central nervous system (CNS) depression in the baby

PARACERVICAL BLOCK

This form of anesthesia is injected by way of the vagina into the cervical region and is effective within five minutes of administration. Paracervical block is rarely used for labor as a result of its association with fetal bradycardia, or low heart rate.

The advantage of paracervical block is

◆ Pain relief during first stage labor with unimpaired ability to bear down during the second stage

The disadvantages of paracervical block are

◆ Depressed labor contractions
◆ An almost invariable use of electronic fetal monitoring
◆ Bradycardia in the baby
◆ Depression of the baby's central nervous system
◆ A risk of the drug's being injected into the baby causing seizure or vascular collapse

PUDENDAL BLOCK

This form of regional anesthesia is administered through the vagina. It blocks sensation around the vaginal area and takes effect within two to five minutes. Pudendal block also facilitates the use of forceps or vacuum extraction and eliminates pain during episiotomy or laceration repair.

The advantage of pudendal block is

◆ Pain relief during second-stage labor

The disadvantages of pudendal block are

◆ Possible elimination of the urge to push
◆ Hematoma
◆ Incidence of infection
◆ Possible CNS depression in the baby

OXYTOCIC DRUGS

A few mothers have on-and-off contractions for several days before labor becomes active. Sometimes labor takes a pause, like a hiker stopping for a rest midway up the mountain. This pause doesn't mean that labor is petering out or somehow abnormal. It is just the way some labors unfold. Sometimes the cause of a stopped labor is physical. Emotional factors, however, can also cause labor to slow down or stop, because labor is a psychophysiological process readily influenced by emotional factors.

Furthermore, it is often the hospital staff and policies that *cause* labor to slow down. Everyone knows a watched pot doesn't boil. When nurses or physicians stand about waiting for labor to become active, the laboring woman often becomes anxious, wondering if her body is indeed performing correctly. The very pressure to perform can impair labor, which is, as we have seen, a mind-body process readily influenced by emotional factors.

Furthermore, in many hospitals labor is expected to progress within a certain time frame. If the laboring woman does not make progress within that time, her labor is augmented with intravenous Pitocin, an artificial form of the pituitary hormone oxytocin, which helps to regulate uterine contractions. Pitocin may be recommended when labor does not progress on its own and there is no other way to get it going.

The advantage of Pitocin is that

◆ It augments or induces labor contractions.

The disadvantages of Pitocin are

◆ Labor contractions tend to be more painful.
◆ Contractions are usually more tumultuous, less easy to manage; contractions seem to rise suddenly to a peak rather than building gradually.
◆ The risk of cesarean surgery is greatly increased.
◆ Electronic fetal monitoring is "required."
◆ The risk of newborn jaundice (and possibly death[19]) is greater.

Alternatives to Pitocin

Unless there are medical complications, *all* of the alternatives should be tried before Pitocin is used. Bear in mind that using medication to augment a slowed labor is often a case of repairing something that's already working fine, only to have it really break down. Use of oxytocic drugs is frequently the first step in an obstetrical round-robin. It goes like this: A woman's labor stops or slows down—frequently as a result of being admitted to a frightening, impersonal environment. Pitocin is administered to augment contractions. This causes more painful contractions. The laboring woman requires medication. The medication further slows labor. The Pitocin dosage is increased. And on and on until fetal distress is recorded on the monitor and the decision to do an "*emergency*" cesarean is made. (Of course, the mother will feel grateful that the cesarean was able to "*save*" her baby. Ironically, if she hadn't given birth in a technically-oriented setting, the baby would probably not have experienced distress in the first place.)

Several studies have shown that disturbance in the birth place impairs labor and even affects the health of the offspring. Other factors that can prolong labor include tension between the laboring woman and her birth partner, the presence of someone with whom she feels uncomfortable, physical inhibitions, and strong negative feelings about becoming a mother. Labor can often be augmented without drugs by meeting the mother's psychological needs through counseling prior to the birth. If the mother is relaxed, secure, and in a peaceful environment where she is receiving ample emotional support and knows what to expect, she is often better able to labor more rapidly.

Other ways to speed labor include nipple stimulation, love-making (no intercourse if membranes have been ruptured), guided imagery, and walking. Medicinal remedies include homeopathic caulophyllum or cimicifuga (to be used only as recommended by a qualified herbalist or homeopath).

Second-Stage Labor

PUSHING

Breathe and push in harmony with your body's needs. When you breathe with your body's urge, you probably won't hold your breath to help you push during labor. Nevertheless, in a few conventional hospitals mothers are enthusiastically coached to take a breath, hold it, and push while a nurse or a group of nurses does a countdown from five or ten to zero. Holding your breath while pushing can cause a decreased supply of oxygen to your baby and increase your chance of having a perineal laceration.

Some hospitals and physicians set arbitrary time limits on how long the mother should push before medical intervention begins. This is an absurdity since every woman's labor is different and her pushing time may last from ten minutes to four hours. At one time prolonged pushing (greater than two and a half hours) was thought to be related to poorer fetal well-being, increased infection for the mother, and postpartum hemorrhage. Recent research, however, has challenged the need to adhere to such arbitrary time limits for second-stage labor.

EPISIOTOMY

Avoid an episiotomy unless there are such medical complications as fetal distress or shoulder dystocia (in which the shoulders get stuck during birth). An episiotomy is perhaps justified if the baby is distressed or in an unusual position, as it facilitates the birth. However, many conventional physicians cut an episiotomy on every mother. They argue that it shortens the birth process and substitutes a neat, easier-to-repair cut for a jagged tear. As neat as it may be, the episiotomy is usually far *larger* than most natural tears and more painful during the postpartum period. For that matter, if you take the steps recommended below, it is likely that you will not tear at all.

An extensive search of the medical literature reveals no support for the routine episiotomies performed by the majority of U.S. obstetricians.[20] In the Netherlands, a country with much less focus on medical intervention during childbirth than the United States and a much lower incidence of infant mortality, the rate of episiotomy is 6 percent, compared to close to 90 percent in the United States.

Alternatives to Episiotomy

Many physicians and midwives now do episiotomies only rarely, if at all. They are skilled at manipulating the perineal tissue over the baby's head and will use perineal massage or hot compresses to help the woman avoid tearing. Even more important, they have learned to trust the mother's body to give birth without unnecessary surgery.

Your birth partner, friend, or childbirth companion can do perineal massage. The Association of Childbirth Companions requires all labor support providers to learn it as part of the training program. Perineal massage during contractions in late first-stage and second-stage labor increases circulation to the perineal area; makes the tissue more supple, reducing the chance of tearing; and relaxes the perineal musculature.

To perform the massage, be sure your hands are clean. Insert your first two fingers knuckle-deep inside the vagina. Make smooth semicircles, pressing downward gently and firmly. Ask the mother if this is comfortable for her, and adjust the pressure as she wishes. Use oil if desired. Vitamin E oil is popular with midwives.

Alternate massaging with applying hot compresses to the perineum. When you can see the baby's head in the birth outlet, be sure to remind the mother to touch it! For many women, this is a magical moment.

Postpartum Procedures

Routine separation of mother and baby during the hours that follow birth has to be one of the most bizarre customs of modern times. For that matter, if you were to make a list of the most bizarre customs in anthropological history, this would be at the top of the list.

In a few hospitals, the newborn is taken to a central nursery, where she usually shrieks at the top of her lungs, and the mother is taken to a recovery room where—if she is not in a drugged stupor—she almost invariably worries about her child.

Animal breeders wouldn't think of handling a birth in such a manner. They don't separate animal mothers and babies, because they know it would have long-term detrimental effects on both. If animal mothers are separated from their young for as short a time as one to four hours during this sensitive period, the mother often fails to provide for her young.

Physicians are just beginning to learn what farmers have known for centuries. Pioneer researchers Drs. Marshall Klaus and John Kennel, who published the results of their ground-breaking research on the subject of maternal-infant attachment, have called attention to the fact that the immediate postpartum period is a very sensitive time for *bonding*, that is, the development of parent-infant attachment.[21] A study conducted at Duke University in North Carolina showed that the breastfeeding rate increased over 50 percent when mothers had no option but to room-in with their infants.[22] Infants who had immediate postnatal contact with their mothers tended to have fewer infections for the first year, gain more weight, and be breastfed longer.[23]

Why is this so? Your baby is especially alert for an hour or so after a natural birth. The mother and father take in and receive their child. By contrast, separation of mothers and infants may lead to temporary or even long-term difficulties in the mother-child relationship.

In one study comparing couples planning home birth, natural hospital birth, and anesthetized hospital delivery, psychotherapist Gayle Peterson and her associates showed that parent-infant attachment seemed to be enhanced by home birth.[24] Again, this is probably because mother and baby are not interrupted.

Research has also revealed that mothers who have prolonged contact with their infants shortly after birth demonstrate greater affection for and attachment to their babies later on. Similarly, a greater percentage of neglect, abuse, and failure to thrive has been found among infants who are separated from their parents shortly after birth. Such dysfunction can be the result of unnatural hospital practices—including routine mother-infant separation and separation of the mother from her family—that have seriously interfered with the parental-infant attachment process.[25]

Fortunately, mother-infant separation (except in medical emergencies requiring immediate pediatric attention) is becoming nothing more than a bad memory as more and more health professionals realize how detrimental it is to the entire family. Keep in mind as well that although this sensitive postbirth period should not be interrupted unless necessary, love can't be reduced to a series of biological patterns. If you aren't able to spend the first postnatal hour with your child for any reason, you will still develop parent-infant attachment.

Following are some instructions for creating an appropriate postpartum setting: *Dim the lights after birth.* Though bright light may sometimes be necessary to examine the baby's color for a few seconds, the room should otherwise be dimly lit. Leaving the womb is probably like stepping out of a low-lit room into a sunny outdoors: the blinding light hurts, and the baby's eyes screw shut in reflex.

If the lighting is low, the baby will open her eyes, look around, and usually lock eyes with the mother and father. That first moment of eye contact can be magical. For me, waves of nameless feeling swept up and down my spine when I first locked eyes with my newborn son.

Remain with your child during all pediatric medical procedures. These include weighing, measuring, applying eye drops to prevent gonococcal infection, and possibly administering vitamin K, as well as taking a blood sample for routine tests.

Delay all nonemergency pediatric procedures for at least one hour while you and your newborn get to know one another. Both mother and father can hold the baby. I usually recommend that the father remove his shirt and hold his newborn against his bare chest for a few minutes, covering the baby's back with a blanket for warmth. This skin-to-skin contact enriches the father's birth experience.

POSTPARTUM BREASTFEEDING

Breastfeed spontaneously and as the baby desires throughout your postpartum period. Immediate postbirth breastfeeding is practically the rule for most contemporary mothers. It is common knowledge that breast milk provides far better nutrition than formula for premature as well as full-term babies. In addition to meeting all the infant's nutritional needs, breast milk protects the baby against many allergies and diseases. The premilk substance called *colostrum* helps the baby to clear excess mucus from the mouth and throat while supplying antibodies to a host of diseases, particularly of the intestinal tract. Another advantage of breast-feeding is that when the baby sucks the breast, the pituitary gland releases the hormone oxytocin, which causes the uterus to contract, thereby facilitating the delivery of the placenta and helping to prevent postpartum hemorrhage. And finally, breastfeeding has been shown to have long-term psychological benefits for the child.

Yet in a few hospitals, certain practices are detrimental to breastfeeding. For example, babies are often placed in a central nursery, separated from the mother. There the baby is frequently given water or formula, which interferes with the breastfeeding pattern. Many maternity nurses use alcohol wash, which can cause the mother's nipples to dry, crack, and bleed. When the mothers breastfeed, it can be painful. Avoid these customs if they are practiced in your area.

Relieving Baby Blues

If you include all your maternity care options in your birth plan, you are more likely to have a healthier, happier adjustment to new parenthood. Many, if not the majority, of American mothers suffer some form of *baby blues*—a constellation of tears, irritability, and depression that begins about the third to fifth day after birth and continues for a period of anywhere from a couple of days to several weeks. I have heard childbirth educators tell parents that baby blues are a normal, almost inevitable part of childbearing.

This is incorrect.

While fluctuating emotions are natural after having a baby, baby blues don't have to be inevitable. Conventional hospital practices contribute to the baby blues. According to Helen Varney of the maternal-newborn program at Yale University's School of Nursing, "Postpartum blues are largely a psychological phe-nomenon of the woman who is separated from her family and her baby."[26] The blues are less common when unnatural birth customs are avoided. British pediatrician Aidan MacFarlane reports that depression occurs in about 60 percent of mothers who give birth in hospitals but only 16 percent of mothers who give birth at home.[27]

There are probably a couple of reasons for this. First, at home mother and baby are not separated during the sensitive period immediately following birth. Second, in the home—as in child-bearing centers and an increasing number of hospitals—you make the most natural transition to becoming a mother. You are not separated from your family. Avoiding prolonged separation of the new mother and her family can mean a healthier adjustment for everyone.

Cesarean Birth

Every birth options plan should include:

◆ Steps to prevent cesarean surgery both during pregnancy and during labor

◆ Contingency plans on the off chance that a cesarean becomes necessary despite your best efforts to avoid the surgery

Never before in the history of childbirth have expectant mothers faced the high risk they do today of surgical birth. Since the 1960s the cesarean rate has more than quadrupled. The U.S. cesarean rate—one of the world's highest—is 27 percent.[1] That means one out of four mothers gives birth via major abdominal surgery. By comparison, in the Netherlands the cesarean rate is about 7 percent.

In some U.S. and Canadian hospitals, the cesarean rate is even higher—30 or even 40 percent! Horrifying as it may seem, the overwhelming majority of cesarean births are unnecessary and avoidable.[2] Most cesareans are *iatrogenic*, that is, doctor-caused. They often result from injudicious use of medical procedures, from electronic fetal monitoring to Pitocin.[3] Ironically, most physicians readily admit the cesarean rate is too high. Nevertheless, physicians and hospitals continue to overuse the medical intervention that increases the cesarean rate.

Therefore it is up to you—the health care consumer—to

decrease your own cesarean rate by creating a birth options plan with cesarean preventive measures.

Surgical Birth Trauma

Cesarean surgery is associated with a constellation of physical and emotional problems that I call surgical birth trauma. Elements of the trauma, which affects the entire family, are:

♦ The unique physical problems of the cesarean mother. These include a slightly higher risk of maternal mortality, more postpartum illness (particularly infection), increased risk of hemorrhage, injury to adjacent organs during the operation, aspiration pneumonia, postoperative gas pains, and a far longer, more uncomfortable postpartum recovery period.

♦ Mother-infant separation and its consequences.

♦ The emotional consequences of cesarean birth for both parents. Parents may feel grief, disappointment, frustration, guilt, feelings of inadequacy, and a sense of failure. Postcesarean emotions vary from one mother to another. For some, negative feelings may last months, even years after the operation.

♦ The unique physical problems of the cesarean-born baby. These include an increased risk of respiratory distress syndrome and jaundice.

Preventing an Unnecessary Cesarean

The mother who gives birth in a childbearing center or at home, or who is attended by a midwife, has a far lower chance of unnecessary surgery than the mother who plans a conventional hospital birth or who is transferred to a hospital. For example, a recent study of childbearing centers nationwide showed the cesarean rate to be 4 percent—less than one-sixth our national average. If you do opt for hospital birth, however, you can still lower your chance of a cesarean by following *all* the steps below.

Pregnancy

◆ Eat a healthy, well-balanced diet.

◆ Exercise regularly.

◆ Examine your beliefs about childbirth.

◆ Develop a positive attitude about childbirth.

◆ Plan your birth carefully.

◆ Choose a competent maternity health care provider with a low cesarean rate and with whom both parents are psychologically compatible.

◆ Choose a birth place with a low cesarean rate and an emotionally positive climate.

◆ Prepare to have effective labor support.

Labor

◆ Have continual support through labor.

◆ Eat and drink to satisfy your body's desires.

◆ Take warm showers and baths as you wish.

◆ Walk around as much as you want.

◆ Adopt the position that is most comfortable for you and change position as you want.

◆ Avoid setting time limits. Allow labor to unfold in its own natural rhythm.

◆ Express yourself freely and without inhibition.

◆ Use guided imagery to help you relax and cope with labor. Use guided imagery to enhance labor's progress, if necessary.

◆ Avoid all medical intervention unless there are genuine complications.

◆ Avoid hormonal augmentation of labor until you have tried all other means of enhancing labor's progress.

Vaginal Birth After a Previous Cesarean

Mothers who have had cesareans often wonder if they can give birth to their next child vaginally. Not long ago physicians frowned upon vaginal birth after a previous cesarean (VBAC). VBAC was so outside the mainstream that many mothers had (and some still have) difficulty finding a health care provider who would help them with VBAC. Today, however, we know that VBACs are safer than repeat cesareans for most women (depending on the type of previous uterine scar and other factors). The medical profession is slowly coming to accept VBAC as the standard of care for previous cesarean mothers. Innumerable studies have proven that the overwhelming majority of repeat cesareans, which make up 35 percent of all cesareans in the United States, are avoidable.

The VBAC mother is at higher risk of cesarean surgery, but not because of any physical abnormality. Rather the high risk stems from two causes: Most VBAC mothers have strong emotions about their prior cesarean that can influence their future labor. If that is your situation, you should spend time preparing prenatally for birth without surgery discussed ahead. In addition, the VBAC mother is at greater risk of iatrogenic surgery—surgery brought on by medical treatment. It is therefore essential to select a physician or midwife with a cesarean rate of less than 10 percent who wholly supports VBAC.

BENEFITS OF VAGINAL BIRTH AFTER A PREVIOUS CESAREAN

With very few exceptions, it is usually better to opt for a vaginal birth rather than a repeat cesarean. Following are some advantages associated with VBAC:

♦ Less likelihood of postpartum illness. Postpartum infection is far less common in mothers who deliver vaginally than in those who have elective repeat cesareans.

♦ Less likelihood of postpartum depression.

♦ A much smoother, easier postpartum period. Caring for the new baby, breastfeeding, and adjusting to motherhood are far easier after a vaginal birth than after an operation, when the mother is in need of medical care.

♦ A safer birth for mother and baby. Vaginal birth carries a much lower risk of maternal or infant mortality than repeat cesarean.

◆ No chance of iatrogenic (doctor-caused) prematurity. Respiratory distress resulting from cesarean delivery is a primary cause of perinatal death. Babies delivered by elective cesarean often require respiratory support even if they are not premature.

◆ A better beginning for the new family. Mother, father, siblings, and new baby are more likely to be happy and psychologically healthy after a normal birth.

◆ Shorter or no time in the hospital.

◆ Decreased cost. Vaginal birth is far less expensive than cesarean surgery.

Preparing for Your VBAC

Your chances of giving birth naturally after a cesarean are just as good as those of the woman who has never given birth, if there are no problems in *this* pregnancy and your cesarean was for a reason unlikely to recur. Many cesareans are done for such reasons as the breech position and fetal distress. Recurrent causes include mental illness or severe pelvic contraction. CPD (cephalopelvic disproportion: a condition in which the baby's head is thought to be too large for the mother's pelvis) is not a recurrent reason.

One study showed a 89 percent VBAC rate among selected patients. In a study conducted by Drs. Richard Meier and Paul Porreco at Kaiser Foundation Hospital in San Diego, out of 207 mothers who had previously had cesareans, 84.5 percent gave birth vaginally. The repeat cesarean rate among these women was therefore 15.5 percent. This is lower than the national cesarean rate (22.7 percent) for all women. Many other studies have shown similar results.

"Everything happened so fast, I lost track of my contractions," recalls Karen about her vaginal birth of her son Brian. A sudden incidence of fetal distress had almost led to another cesarean. However, within a short time she went to full dilation and was pushing. "It was painful. Although it was rough, I was really glad that I had a VBAC." Even if problems should arise and you end with a necessary cesarean, the baby will benefit from labor and have less chance of respiratory distress. And you and your partner will feel you've done the best you possibly could. This confidence will greatly reduce the effects of surgical birth trauma.

To increase your likelihood of a safe, rewarding vaginal birth, observe the following:

- If you haven't experienced labor, learn about it. You should have a realistic idea of labor's pain and prepare yourself with effective coping methods (strong labor support, guided imagery, and perhaps rhythmic breathing patterns).

- Choose a health care provider who will treat you as if you haven't had a cesarean. It is not sufficient if your health care provider is willing to allow a "trial of labor." Many claim to support VBAC yet treat the mother as if she were planning to give birth while skydiving.

- If you are mistrustful of your prior health care provider and you believe the cesarean was unnecessary, find a more supportive health care provider for this birth.

- If you plan a hospital birth, be sure the hospital you choose supports vaginal birth after a prior cesarean—and not in name only. Meet the staff and get a feeling for their attitude. The staff of some hospitals recognize that the mother with a prior cesarean has as much likelihood of giving birth safely and normally as everyone else. Yet in a few hospitals insensitive staff persons are hostile to VBAC mothers.

- Arrange for effective, continuous labor support. VBAC mothers need support even more than women who are laboring for the first time, because they tend to be more anxious.

- Consider hiring a childbirth companion, unless the father is wholly committed to learning about effective support during pregnancy and being actively involved throughout labor.

- Use all nonpharmacologic forms of pain relief before resorting to pain medication.

- If you have an electronic fetal monitor, use it only intermittently so that you can be up and walking.

IS THE INCISION SAFE?

There are two types of abdominal incisions used for cesarean surgery. The most common is the *pfannenstiel incision*. It is a horizontal cut above the pubic hairline. The *midline incision* is faster to cut and is used in rare emergencies when speed is an issue. It is a vertical incision running from a little below the navel to just below the pubic hairline.

The abdominal incision does not indicate the type of *uterine incision*. It is the uterine incision that should be considered when planning a normal birth after a cesarean.

There are three different types of uterine incisions used for surgical birth. The *low transverse*, sometimes called *low segment* or *Kerr*, incision is the most common and most preferred method of cesarean delivery under ordinary circumstances. The low transverse is a horizontal incision in the lower part of the uterus near the cervix. It is used in over 90 percent of cesareans today.

The *low vertical* or *Kroenig* incision is used rarely, in cases of unusual presentations or if the baby is very large or very small. Risk of rupture is greater, since no one can be sure how much of the uterus is incised.

The once-common *classic* incision is sometimes used for unusual presentations or if the placenta covers the uterine segment. This is the incision associated with the greatest risk among VBAC mothers.

The type of uterine scar you have is included in your medical records. If you are currently visiting a new health care provider, your records should be routinely requested.

THE VBAC MOTHER'S SPECIAL NEEDS

The overwhelming majority of cesarean mothers planning a vaginal birth are perfectly normal. You are, however, in a special situation. If healthy first-time laboring women are sometimes treated like invalids in America, you can imagine how the woman who has had a prior cesarean is often treated, despite the fact that she is as healthy as anyone else.

The term used to describe labor after a previous cesarean— "trial of labor"—may increase the VBAC mother's anxiety. You may wonder whether your so-called trial of labor will be successful.

Many parents fear uterine rupture. Though there is hardly any risk of scar separation, and the risk is the same as it is with elective repeat cesarean, it is nonetheless a real fear.

The *routine* procedure for VBAC at one particular hospital I've heard about is as follows: The woman is immediately hooked up to EFM on arrival. Intravenous infusion is begun. The mother is restricted from eating or drinking and advised to eat small amounts of ice chips. She is fed an antacid every three to four hours to neutralize stomach acidity. Supplies are placed right in her room in case of an emergency. These include a catheter, urinary drainage bag, and an abdominal prep kit (for preoperative procedures). When membranes rupture, internal electronic fetal monitoring is begun. With a setup like this, it is a wonder that any so-called trials of labor succeed!

Understanding the following facts will help you better plan your birth:

◆ The VBAC mother is at greater risk of medical intervention. You and your baby should be watched diligently to be sure everything is progressing normally. However, this can be done without making you feel as if you were hovering on the brink of disaster. You should not have to submit to unnecessary intervention, nor should you be treated like a high-risk patient because of something that happened perhaps several years ago. Injudicious medical intervention increases the risk of repeat cesarean. Once again, choose your health care provider and birth place carefully.

◆ The VBAC mother needs to develop confidence and a positive view of birth even more than the woman who hasn't given birth previously. Many expectant parents lack confidence in the body's ability to give birth naturally. Frequently this is especially true of those who have had prior cesareans. The mother with a prior cesarean can learn to trust her body. It helps if the father learns as much as he can about birth and develops confidence in his ability to support his partner effectively. You can develop confidence in several ways. Talk to a health care provider or childbirth educator. Share your feelings with other VBAC and cesarean parents. Consider joining a support group, such as ICAN, a cesarean support group with branches nationwide.

◆ The VBAC parent frequently needs to work out unresolved feelings about her prior birth. Many mothers planning a VBAC have strong negative feelings about their cesarean. If these feelings remain unresolved, they can interfere with the present labor and make you and your partner mistrustful of your current health care providers. Therefore, expressing your concerns, anger, frustration, and perhaps grief over your past cesarean is essential. Many parents find themselves confronting a flood of tears years after the event. Releasing your feelings and forgiving those involved will open the door for healing.

Your chance of delivering vaginally is slightly reduced if you have had a cesarean for CPD. However, it is still excellent. Many studies have proven that the overwhelming majority of mothers previously sectioned for CPD may still give birth normally. In an exhaustive study by Drs. Meier and Porreco, 78 percent of mothers who initially had cesareans because of failure to progress in labor for CPD subsequently gave birth vaginally. In another study by Dr. Richard Paul and his associates at the Los Angeles County–University of Southern California Medical Center at Women's Hospital, 77 percent of mothers who previously had cesareans for CPD gave birth vaginally.[4] The rate of uterine dehiscence in this study was no higher among VBAC mothers than among those who had planned cesareans. Often the babies who are born vaginally are as large or larger than those for which the mother previously had a cesarean.

When a Cesarean Birth Is Necessary

Though you should try to avoid surgical birth, a cesarean is occasionally necessary to preserve the health of the mother or baby. Under the following conditions a cesarean section is recommended:

◆ Placental abruption (all or part of the placenta separates from the uterine wall). If the abruption is complete, a cesarean is performed to prevent maternal hemorrhage and fetal death.

◆ Placenta previa (the placenta covers all or part of the cervix at the time of birth). A cesarean is performed to prevent severe maternal blood loss and fetal death.

◆ Umbilical cord prolapse (the umbilical cord precedes the baby in the birth canal). In this condition, the baby's oxygen supply is cut off and a cesarean is usually necessary to prevent brain damage or death from asphyxia.

◆ Malpresentation (the baby is in other than the vertex, or head-down, position). In the breech position (buttocks or feet first in the birth canal), the baby can often be delivered vaginally, though this position is associated with complications. The baby in the transverse lie (shoulders first in the birth canal) cannot be delivered vaginally.

◆ An active case of genital herpes. While passing through the canal, the baby can become infected, leading to permanent damage or death.

◆ Diabetes mellitus. Mothers with this condition run a higher risk of fetal death during the last few weeks of pregnancy. Accordingly, a preterm cesarean is often done if the condition is severe.

◆ Other maternal illnesses. A few illnesses contribute to serious complications for either mother or baby. These include preeclampsia/eclampsia (a pregnancy disease characterized by hypertension, swelling, and protein in the urine); chronic hypertension (high blood pressure); and certain cardiac and kidney diseases.

If you have one of these conditions at the time of giving birth, you may need cesarean surgery. Whether you plan surgery in advance or the physician makes the decision at the last minute during labor, you can take the simple steps discussed below to make your birth a joyful event and your postcesarean recovery as smooth as possible. They will reduce the surgical birth trauma for the entire family. Besides, you will have done all you could to avoid *unnecessary* surgical birth.

You can also reduce surgical birth trauma by making informed decisions, remaining with your partner throughout your experience, being as active a participant as possible under the circumstances, prolonging parent-infant contact directly following delivery, breastfeeding immediately or as soon after birth as possible, and arranging for the help of family or friends during your postpartum recovery.

You have choices that influence your cesarean birth experience and postpartum recovery. Rarely is there a life-threatening situation when medical experts must make decisions so rapidly that there is no time for the mother and father to have input.

The most important choices regard:

◆ Type of anesthesia

◆ How the father will be involved during surgery and immediately afterward

◆ Parent-infant contact after birth

Making informed decisions about these issues will help reduce surgical birth trauma.

ANESTHESIA FOR CESAREAN BIRTH

Physicians use two basic types of anesthesia for cesarean surgery: *general anesthesia*, in which the mother is unconscious, and *regional anesthesia*, in which the mother is anesthetized but conscious for the birth. In addition, local anesthesia and acupuncture have rarely been used.

General anesthesia is occasionally used in emergencies when speed is essential to save the life of mother or baby, as, for example, in the severe case of placenta previa involving massive maternal bleeding. Some low-back problems, certain allergies, and hypotension (low blood pressure) may also contraindicate the use of regional anesthesia. In addition, some women choose general because they would rather not be awake during the operation.

When it is time to administer the anesthetic, Pentothal sodium is added to the IV. It then takes only fifteen to twenty seconds for the mother to become unconscious. Once she is unconscious, the anesthesiologist passes a tube down the throat and into the windpipe to prevent aspiration of stomach contents. (This procedure, called endotracheal intubation, sometimes causes a mild sore throat for a few days.) Nitrous oxide and oxygen are then given to maintain the anesthesia. The mother wakes up when the surgery is completed.

The major disadvantage is the very slight risk of aspirating stomach contents, possibly leading to severe pneumonia. Other disadvantages are that the mother is not awake for the birth and mother and baby are too groggy to participate in the bonding process for several hours afterward.

In most hospitals the father and childbirth companion are not permitted in the delivery room when general anesthesia is used. However, some hospitals and physicians will make an exception.

Regional anesthesia includes both spinal and epidural. Both numb the body from the chest to the toes and render the area temporarily immobile.

Most cesarean mothers prefer regional anesthesia so they can be awake to experience the birth and see the baby immediately afterward. Several studies have shown that mothers who had regional anesthesia tend to have more positive perceptions of their cesarean experience than those who had general.

With regional anesthesia, you may feel pressure, tugging, and pulling sensations during surgery, but there should be no pain. If you do feel pain, simply tell the physician so he or she can adjust the anesthesia.

For both spinal and epidural, the mother lies on her side with her back curled toward the anesthesiologist. The spinal involves only a single injection. Spinals are sometimes followed by spinal headaches requiring the mother to remain flat on her back for eight hours or so. These may be the result of the leakage of a small quantity of cerebrospinal fluid through the puncture holes. Spinal headaches have become less common since the introduction of small-gauge needles to administer the anesthetic.

Most consider epidural the anesthesia of choice for a cesarean because there is less risk of aftereffects and it is easier to control. A very thin, hollow tube is inserted into the back and taped in place for the duration of the surgery. This way, more anesthetic can be injected as needed.

Occasionally, there is a *window*, that is, an area not fully anesthetized. However, this is rare, and if it does occur, the anesthesiologist can adjust the anesthetic.

THE BIRTH

A cesarean section generally takes about an hour in total. The baby is usually born within the first fifteen minutes. The remaining time is spent stitching the incisions.

Although you and your partner are bound to feel anything but relaxed, there is usually plenty of time to ask questions and make informed decisions. However, in extreme emergencies (such as severe placental abruption or a prolapsed cord) the procedure is speeded up.

The following procedures are done shortly before surgery, usually in the labor room: The abdomen is shaved. An IV is started, and a catheter is inserted through the urethra into the bladder to remove fluid from the bladder. Antacid is given to neutralize stomach acids.

In many hospitals, mothers are routinely given sedation. This causes grogginess during and after the birth for both mother and baby. If you prefer to be fully alert, request no preoperative medication.

When you are moved to the delivery room and onto the delivery table, routine procedures generally include strapping the arms to two boards extended on either side of the table (like the wings of an airplane) or to your sides. This prevents you from inadvertently touching the sterile area. You can request that one arm be free (or loosely strapped) or that the strap be removed immediately after birth so you can touch your baby.

Sometimes the leads to a cardiac monitor are placed on your chest to give continual heartbeat feedback during the operation. A blood pressure cuff is attached to your arm so your pressure can be checked frequently.

The anesthetic will then be administrated and surgery begun.

The father should be allowed to be present during the preoperative procedures. This is an anxious time, and the mother will benefit from her partner's continual presence and support. If being together without separation is important to you, be sure the hospital permits this. You can discuss this point with your health care provider.

Shortly after surgery is begun, you will see your baby. Ask your physician to show you the baby when she is born. Unless there is an emergency, this should be routine. The baby will then be examined by a nurse or pediatrician; you can request that the exam be done near you so that you can observe it. The baby's nose and throat may have to be suctioned to clear mucus from the air passageways.

After the exam the father should take the baby and hold it close to you. You can caress the infant with your hands or your face, kiss her, smell the fresh odor of the newborn, and enjoy eye-to-eye contact. Also begin breastfeeding as soon as possible.

The baby will keep her eyes closed in a brightly lit delivery room. She has been used to the near-dark womb, and bright light hurts the sensitive newborn eyes. Unfortunately, bright lights are necessary during cesarean surgery. Cupping a hand just above the baby's eyes encourages the infant to open them.

If immediate pediatric care is necessary, the baby is taken to an intensive care unit (ICU). Depending on the parents' preference, the father can either remain with the mother while she's being stitched or accompany the child to the ICU. If he goes to the ICU, he can later share the baby's first actions with the mother. After the mother is stitched, she can also go to the ICU on a rolling bed to see the baby.

From time to time the new parents may need to remind themselves that although cesarean surgery is not what they would have chosen, it is after all an occasion to celebrate. A child is born.

Relieving Postcesarean Discomforts

INCISION DISCOMFORT

The discomfort in the incision area will be much less within a week. Meanwhile the following may help:

- ◆ Pain-relief medication. This is the most effective remedy. Don't worry about the medication reaching the baby if you are breastfeeding. The amount that reaches the baby is minimal.

◆ The guided imagery exercise called *The Radiant Breath* to promote healing. Imagine as you breathe in that the breath is a soft, golden, radiant light. Breathe this light into the area of discomfort and imagine the light healing the area.

◆ Using either the side-lying position or the football hold while breastfeeding. Or sit up with a pillow over the incision.

GAS PAIN

For most cesarean mothers gas pain, ranging from mild to severe, is the major discomfort. Because of both anesthesia and the surgical procedure, bowel function is delayed for a while. Excess gas may build up as the intestines start to work by the second or third postpartum day. The gas buildup is actually a positive sign that things are getting back to normal.

The following measures may help relieve the pain:

◆ Rock in a rocking chair while nursing your baby. Intervals of rocking help many cesarean mothers prevent or reduce gas pain.

◆ Avoid carbonated beverages, apple juice (which can be gas-producing), iced drinks (ice chips, however, are fine), and drinking through a straw (which can increase air intake). Avoid any other foods that normally cause you to form gas.

◆ Move about in bed often. Roll from side to side.

◆ Walk frequently.

◆ Do abdominal tightening.

◆ Lie on your left side, draw up your knees, and massage your abdomen from right to left.

◆ Try the medicinal remedies hot fennel, peppermint, or ginger tea.

If the discomfort is severe and none of these methods relieve it, tell your health care provider or a nurse. Sometimes a thin tube can be placed in the rectum to relieve the gas. This is not painful.

SHOULDER PAIN

Many postcesarean mothers experience pain in one or both shoulders. This is caused by blood or air collecting under the diaphragm. The pain is deferred through nerve passages to the shoulder. It passes in two or three days. Medication prescribed by the physician is the most effective relief.

Midwifery Care

Donna and Karl, both clinical psychologists in New Jersey, were so committed to midwifery care that it was either a midwife or no attendant. In Donna's words, "I didn't want to relinquish control over such an intensely personal event in Karl's and my life. We intended to birth our baby with people who respected our needs and intelligence." During labor, with her husband and midwife to support her, Donna recalls "feeling encircled with love and safety."

Thousands of parents have had similar experiences. Midwives are becoming the health care providers of choice for more parents every day.

Throughout history midwives have played a prominent role in the lives of families. "It is the oldest honorable profession," says Janet Tipton,. a midwife in East Texas. People throughout the world respected and honored midwives. However, the past two centuries brought dramatic changes. Midwifery fell into disrepute in Europe. The United States virtually eradicated midwives. Today the trend is being reversed. Midwives are again rising in popularity. The number of hospital births attended by midwives has increased five-fold from 1975 to 1987 and continues to grow. Midwife-attended home birth is seeing a similar jump.

The near death of the world's most ancient health profession is one of the strangest and darkest chapters in childbirth history. As early as the eighteenth century, "male midwives" (an old name for doctors who provided obstetric care) became fashionable. Despite initial cultural resistance, women—particularly middle- and upper-class women—came to prefer the male midwives because they

118

appeared to have more thorough medical knowledge. It was childbearing women who originally made the choice that initiated the horror to come. This fact bears serious thought. Health care consumers create the conditions of their own birth experience just as health care consumers are responsible for making change.

Once established, physicians in Europe and America began to wage a bitter campaign to defame and devalue traditional midwives. Midwives, who worked independently of one another, lacked organization, leadership, and educational programs (though there were a few midwifery schools dating from the sixteenth century). As a result, though experience and skills varied from one midwife to another, many midwives' practices became outdated while the medical profession continued to advance. In addition, the lack of license requirements and formal supervision kept midwives from being officially recognized as part of the health care system.

Physicians brought both great advances and dire perils to childbirth. On the positive side, they made midwifery a science, the forerunner of obstetrics. Doctors established programs of education, published books, and developed technological interventions to help women in childbirth when nature failed.

However, as doctors replaced the midwives, a pattern developed that health care consumers are only now beginning to reverse. As in more recent times, physicians overused medical procedures, sometimes causing illness and death. Under the physician's care, birth became less of a social event shared by the family. Worse, doctors introduced the most gruesome chapter in the history of childbirth: puerperal fever. During the nineteenth century, puerperal or "childbed" fever, a severe and often fatal infection, reached epidemic proportions, killing thousands of new mothers. Doctors created this terrible tragedy by failing to wash their hands after examining cadavers or ill patients and before doing vaginal exams. Doctors and nurses carried the infection from one mother to another. Most women who chose to give birth at home—and even those who accidentally gave birth on the hospital steps or in the corridors, on their way to the maternity wards— were spared. The infection raged until the latter part of the nineteenth century, when antiseptic hand washing became standard practice.

Nowhere on earth did midwifery come as close to being

eradicated as in the United States. Midwives were among the first people to settle the colonies. At the turn of the twentieth century, they were still delivering about half the babies. Yet by 1935, midwives were delivering only about 12 percent of babies. The trend toward doctor-managed labor continued until the 1970's when physicians were delivering well over 95 percent of all babies.[1]

While midwives are still fighting for recognition in the United States, they enjoy a far higher status in other developed countries. For example, while midwives still attend little more than 5 percent of births in the United States, they attend nearly three-quarters of the births in Great Britain. Nations with far lower infant mortality rates than the United States, such as the Netherlands, Denmark, and Japan respect midwives. In these countries midwives attend somewhere between 60 and 80 percent of all births.

What Is a Midwife?

A midwife is a person who gives prenatal care, delivers babies, gives postpartum care, provides normal newborn care, and sometimes provides well-woman care.

Midwives are fond of quoting the literal meaning of their title—from the Anglo-Saxon, mid, "with," and wif, "woman." The slogan "Midwife means with woman" is becoming popular in childbirth circles. I've seen it on bumper stickers, cloth tote bags, and T-shirts. It emphasizes the midwife's commitment to working with the mother or, as some put it, "to serving the childbearing woman."

In 1955 the American College of Nurse-Midwives (ACNM) was established to certify members of their profession. Gradually nurse-midwives have become nationally recognized health professionals. They have also formed state, regional, and national networks to promote midwifery care and to work toward the legalization of their practice. In 1982 the Midwives Alliance of North America (MANA) was founded to improve communication among all midwives and to establish guidelines for basic competency and safety. MANA is a member of the International Confederation of Midwives, which sets standards for the practice of midwifery worldwide.

Both men and women practice midwifery. In 1988, however, fewer than one hundred of the four thousand certified nurse-midwives who practiced in the United States were men. Nevertheless, more men are becoming interested in the profession as stereotypes identifying nursing and midwifery as "women's work" crumble.

The qualities that distinguish a good midwife are more important than gender. Most childbirth professionals agree: the ideal midwife should have a thorough background in the anatomy and physiology of pregnancy and labor, recognize complications, work in close collaboration with a backup physician and hospital should a transfer be necessary, and be flexible enough to meet the parents' individual goals. They should also have a nonjudgmental approach and, as one physician put it, "a lot of love in the heart."

Though *midwife* and *midwifery* refer to a specific health profession, these terms also have a broader meaning. More important than whether the health care professional is a physician or midwife is the philosophy of maternity care. The goal for parents and baby is to receive nurturing support without unnecessary medical intervention, no matter who provides that care. One family physician says, "I think of midwifery as a style of practice and I'm honored to have my clients think of me as a midwife." In this sense of the term, a physician, naturopath, or chiropractor, as well as a midwife, can practice midwifery.

TRAINING

Two major types of midwives practice in the United States today: certified nurse-midwives and direct-entry midwives.

Certified Nurse-Midwife (CNM)

A certified nurse-midwife has education in both nursing and midwifery. Being a registered nurse is a prerequisite for nurse-midwifery education. CNMs receive their practical, hands-on experience in a variety of settings, including hospitals, clinics, birth centers, and home birth practices. On completion of the educational program, the midwife receives evidence of certification from the American College of Nurse-Midwives (ACNM), the professional organization for nurse-midwives.

CNMs are well trained. After much clinical experience in teaching hospitals, they are able to give experienced prenatal care, help during childbirth, and recognize complications. They also learn well-woman gynecology and newborn care.

One of my acquaintances, Mary Ellen Doherty, CNM, received her certification from the nurse-midwifery program at New Jersey's University of Medicine and Dentistry. After practicing in Emerson Hospital in Concord, Massachusetts, for a few years, she and two other nurse-midwives opened a private practice, Concord Nurse-Midwifery Associates. The midwives work in collaboration with three backup physicians in case of complications.

Another CNM, Vicky Wolfrum of South Bay Family Care in San Pedro, California, has a unique background. She trained in Switzerland through apprenticeship. She became a registered nurse and began to work in California, a state where lay midwifery is illegal. "You can't keep the clients' best interest at heart if you're worried about breaking the law," she says. So she became a CNM and now attends both home and childbearing center births.

CNMs work in a collaborative relationship with a physician and have physician backup.

Other Midwives

I use the term *direct-entry midwife* to refer to all midwives who are not CNMs, whether they're nurses or not. Internationally this term refers to a person who has completed formal education in midwifery and is licensed or certified to practice in his or her state or province. In the United States, however, the term is often applied to all midwives other than CNMs. Usually this means midwives who have entered the profession "directly," without first having become a nurse. Some nurses, however, have also trained to become midwives without becoming CNMs.

Midwives are hardly in accord about what they should call themselves. During a lunch with a group of midwives who had similar training, I received no less than six different responses from seven women when I asked about the proper name of their profession. One said she thought of herself as an *empirical midwife;* another preferred the term *practical midwife;* a third and fourth liked the term *traditional midwife;* a fifth called herself a *lay midwife;*

Types of Midwives

Several types of midwives of varying backgrounds give prenatal care and attend births.

◆ A *certified nurse-midwife* or CNM (often called simply a nurse-midwife) is educated in both nursing and midwifery according to the requirements of the American College of Nurse-Midwives (ACNM).

◆ A *direct-entry midwife* is often called a midwife, independent midwife, certified or licensed lay midwife, traditional midwife, or empirical midwife. In Europe a direct-entry midwife is one who has been trained in midwifery school with or without prior training in nursing. In the United States this term is often used to refer to a midwife who has entered the profession through some combination of apprenticeship training, midwifery schooling, or a background in nursing.

◆ A *lay midwife* has entered the profession through apprenticeship with an experienced midwife or physician, through midwifery schooling, or a combination of both. Lay midwives have varying levels of skill and experience. In some states midwives are licensed to practice and are regulated by a governing board of health professionals.

◆ A *granny midwife*, most common in the rural South, is a lay midwife helping neighboring women give birth. Most are not formally educated and have no medical background, though they may work closely with public health or medical professionals. Granny midwives are becoming less common.

a sixth, who practiced in New Hampshire, called herself a *licensed midwife;* and the seventh preferred *direct-entry midwife.* After the lunch, I told another midwife about all these terms. She said, "I don't like any of them. I call myself an *independent midwife.*"

Some states, for instance Washington and Arizona, require formal schooling for midwives. Therefore the word *lay* is inappropriate in those states. In other states, such as New Hampshire, *lay* is the officially accepted term.

The background and training of direct-entry midwives can be as varied as their names. Many train through apprenticeship, in midwifery school, or through a combination of the two.

I know several former maternity nurses who have become midwives. Many had extensive experience and witnessed thousands of births before deciding to attend births at home. For example, Lisa Jensen, a midwife practicing in Lyman, New Hampshire, is a registered nurse who trained in midwifery through apprenticeship. Now she is in a community-based nurse-midwifery program, working toward becoming a CNM.

A few midwives train empirically (that is, through experience, often with no academic background in the field). For example, CharLynn Doughtry, who runs the Labor of Love Childbirth Center in Lakeland, Florida, trained empirically through self-study and attending births on her own. "I would tell parents that I was not a midwife," CharLynn recalls, "but I would offer them the experience I had at no charge." She trained this way for five years and is now licensed by the state of Florida.

Another midwife, Joan Remington, founder of the Arizona School of Midwifery, attended her first birth in 1975. "The mother was planning to give birth at home, unattended," she recalls. "Two of us who had given birth previously planned to be with her. The baby was born easily, and mother and baby were perfectly healthy. When I suctioned mucus from the baby's mouth and cut the cord, I realized I had to do more than just attend, believing all would be well. If a problem did develop, I had no skills to handle it. So I decided I would go and get training." Today Joan is a licensed midwife working with a partner, Mary-Ann Baul, in Woman Care Midwifery Associates in Flagstaff, Arizona. They have attended 450 births since 1982 with no infant mortalities.

Direct-entry midwives have varied degrees of skill and experience. They range from highly skilled, qualified, experienced health care providers to persons who claim to be midwives after observing one or two births. Inadequate training is more likely if the midwife's experience comes solely through attending home births as an apprentice. Unless she is in a major city apprenticing for an unusually busy midwife, she would have to spend many years in training to get adequate experience.

MIDWIFERY SCHOOLS

The Dutch, who have one of the world's lowest infant mortality rates, can boast of creating what is probably the ideal system of maternity care—an example I hope the world follows. First, at least 50 percent of mothers give birth at home. Second, in the Netherlands, midwives train in a midwifery school for three years. They observe and participate in hundreds of births, witnessing both complications and normal births.

During the mother's labor, Dutch midwives work with "home helpers," who act much like the childbirth companion in the United States. The home helper trains to help the midwife during labor and to help the mother and infant for ten days after birth. The home helper also does light housekeeping and cooking, besides caring for the mother and baby.

Dutch midwives are not nurses. They are independent professionals with no affiliation with hospitals, nurses, or physicians. They do not have to follow the rules and protocol of other professionals overseeing their activities, but rely on their own professional protocol.

Many direct-entry midwives envision themselves as the American counterparts of the Dutch midwife. Several midwifery schools, such as the Northern Arizona School of Midwifery and the Seattle Midwifery School, provide training in many areas of health care, skill, and study that overlap nursing curriculum.

There are major differences between the Dutch midwife and her American counterpart—differences that make the Dutch system enviably superior. The Dutch midwife is part of an entire national system of medical care. The nation acknowledges, recognizes, and respects her as an integral part of the health care system. In everyone's eyes she is a professional. She provides maternity care in hospitals and at home. In striking contrast, in 1994 the U.S. direct-entry midwife could not officially provide health care in hospitals (though direct-entry midwives are now seeking hospital privileges). In most states the medical establishment does not recognize the direct-entry midwife as a professional.

Some midwifery schools offer thorough instruction for direct-entry midwives. For example, the Seattle Midwifery School, founded in 1978, combines classroom instruction with clinical training supervised by community-based practicing midwives.

Relying on European standards for academic content and clinical experience for direct-entry midwifery programs, the school was the first to successfully pilot comprehensive, professional midwifery training leading to state licensing.

A similar school, the Northern Arizona School of Midwifery in Flagstaff, requires 920 hours of clinical experience besides rigorous academic requirements. The school also requires that midwifery students attend and participate in one hundred prenatal visits, one hundred newborn exams, one hundred postpartum exams, and one hundred births.

Two very busy childbearing centers now offer midwifery training in El Paso: Maternidad La Luz and Casa da Nacimiento. Karen Miller, director of Maternidad La Luz, justifiably refers to El Paso as the "Mecca of midwifery training." No other location in the United States offers so much experience in such a short time. Both schools provide clinical experience at prenatal exams and during labor on site. Students who complete the training then continue apprenticing with other midwives.

Unfortunately, these schools lack ongoing affiliation agreements with hospitals, so most students' experience is limited to home and childbearing center birth. Hopefully this will change as direct-entry midwives become more widely accepted and officially recognized.

The Midwife's View of Birth

Most midwives—CNMs and direct-entry midwives—view birth as a normal, natural process. The majority are committed to providing maternity care with minimal medical intervention. "I had my first baby overseas with nurse-midwives and they were wonderful," says Mary Hammond-Tooke, CNM, of the Maternity Center in Bethesda, Maryland, who attends both home and childbearing center births. "When I came back to the United States, I had the misconception that I would receive better care, since America is so advanced in so many other areas. During my next labor I was appalled at the care I received. The nurses who attended me during labor were not at all helpful. They kept pushing drugs. They didn't understand natural childbirth. After the baby was born, I wasn't allowed to nurse right away. They were not at all supportive of breastfeeding. If I hadn't breastfed the first baby, I would never have breastfed. I decided to become a midwife and help mothers do it differently."

Choosing a midwife does not automatically mean you will receive more nurturing care. Though most midwives embrace a philosophy of noninterventive health care, I have observed midwives who cut episiotomies on every first-time mother and who use electronic fetal monitoring routinely. But the majority of midwives help the mother give birth the way she chooses without unnecessary intervention.

Midwives disagree about who provides better care, CNMs or direct-entry midwives. Many certified nurse-midwives feel that one can't acquire adequate obstetric skills without first becoming a nurse. On the other hand, many direct-entry midwives feel that a nursing background is a hindrance, giving the midwife a medical focus.

Though I personally feel nursing and midwifery should be separate professions, as they are in the Netherlands, many CNMs as well as direct-entry midwives are skilled and highly experienced and also embrace a philosophy of maternity care without unnecessary medical intervention.

PHYSICIANS AND MIDWIVES: THE DIFFERENCE

Though midwives train to recognize complications and handle emergencies, midwifery is the only health profession concerned primarily with a normal, natural event and not an affliction or a disease. As a rule, midwives have a more natural, less medically-oriented approach to childbirth than do physicians.

Bear in mind that this is only a generality. Many obstetricians and family physicians today work with the heart of a midwife, while some midwives work with an overly clinical approach.

One would think that obstetricians with their more advanced education and broader experience would offer better care than midwives. There is no question that obstetricians have more training to handle complications. However, studies suggest that midwives provide safer maternity care during essentially normal pregnancies and labors.

In some ways the midwife's training may actually be superior to the physician's. Many midwives have skills most obstetricians do not. For example, most midwives know how to protect women from tearing by applying warm compresses, doing perineal massage, and gently manipulating the perineum over the baby's head. Peculiar as it may seem, most physicians have not learned these basic skills. Most will cut episiotomies instead.

A few obstetricians are beginning to learn skills from midwives. For example, at a midwifery conference in Baltimore, Maryland, where I was conducting a workshop, two obstetricians had registered to learn skills from a lay-trained midwife.

One important difference between the midwife's and the obstetrician's training is that the midwife has attended many entire labors from beginning to end. In striking contrast, many physicians have never observed even a single labor all the way through: labor experience is a missing ingredient in established obstetrical training. In hospitals nurses, not physicians, take care of laboring women unless there are medical complications requiring the obstetrician's expertise. Physicians learn about labor from studying textbooks and graphs, yet spend only a few minutes with laboring women. In my opinion, this is like learning to fish on dry land.

"You can't learn about labor like that!" exclaims one physician, outraged at the quality of maternity education in obstetrics. "Without listening to every contraction, being right there with a woman, you can't really know labor. You have to be with a woman throughout her labor: ten, twenty-four, thirty-six hours, however long it takes—until the baby is born."

And one can't learn about the experience of labor by studying anatomy and physiology. One can learn about the psychological and emotional changes making up the laboring mind response only from laboring women.

Perhaps the most important difference between the practice of midwives and physicians is that midwives, for the most part, have a better understanding of the experience of labor. Many are consciously or unconsciously aware of the laboring mind response. Understanding how the emotions and mind influence labor allows the midwife to give better maternity care from pregnancy through the postpartum period. This insight into labor may be the reason that, for the most part, midwives have better health statistics than physicians.

Advantages of Midwifery Care

Pioneer obstetrician Richard B. Stewart, founder of the Douglas Birthing Center in Douglasville, Georgia, says, "I firmly believe that the best kind of birth a woman can have is to be attended by a trained midwife, or a doctor who practices like a midwife."

Parents opt to have a midwife attend their birth at home, at a childbearing center, or in a hospital for any or all of the following advantages:

♦ Most midwives are committed to giving noninterventive health care through the childbearing season. The mother who chooses a midwife has a greatly reduced chance of having such intervention as electronic fetal monitoring, intravenous feeding, an episiotomy, and a cesarean section. As Lynn, a California mother put it, "I trusted my body's ability to give birth naturally and didn't want unnecessary medical intervention. So I chose a midwife."

♦ Most midwives spend much more time with clients than physicians do. Most of my midwifery acquaintances allot at least 30 to 60 minutes for each prenatal visit to develop a rapport with the client and better meet her needs.

♦ The midwife remains with the mother throughout labor, or for a significant portion of her labor, providing continuity of care. By contrast, most obstetricians come in at the last minute to deliver the baby. Continuous individual support enables many women to labor more efficiently and feel more secure. Midwives who attend home births or child-bearing center births will often accompany the mother if she transfers to a hospital. The midwife continues to provide support and in some hospitals may provide maternity care.

♦ The mother attended by a midwife has a significantly reduced chance of having an unnecessary cesarean section. "My cervix was so slow to dilate," recalls Carol, a mother in Florida, "that my obstetrician told me that I would have had a cesarean section had I been in the hospital. However, I had chosen a midwife who stayed with me and encouraged me to give birth vaginally."

- Midwives support family-centered care. Most midwives view the father as an intrinsic part of the childbearing experience. Family participation is encouraged if that's what the parents want.

- Midwives provide emotional support as well as physical care. Most midwives help the mother deal with her feelings about becoming a parent and her fears about childbirth. They give her encouragement. This boosts the mother's confidence and often helps her to labor more smoothly.

- Midwives support the parents' individual goals. Most midwives encourage parents to participate actively in their birth. Tom, a father in Florida, says he and his wife found their midwife far more committed to helping them with their last four births than the physician who had provided care during their first birth. "Our first birth was with a doctor," Tom recalls. "He was a wonderful man but only showed up to deliver the baby. He expected us to do everything his way. The midwife was willing to help us give birth the way we wanted and give birth in the place we felt most comfortable, which was our home." "I wasn't happy with my physician," recalls Maggie, a mother of two in Anderson, Indiana. "He wasn't concerned about my needs." She switched to a midwife who was so committed to giving personal care that she changed Maggie's outlook on childbirth. "When I first became pregnant," Maggie goes on, "I wanted a hospital birth with medication, but after talking with my midwife, I felt totally at ease about giving birth naturally."

- Midwives provide care at a cost usually significantly less than that of obstetricians. The midwife's care is usually, but not always, less expensive than the physician's. Occasionally, midwifery care is overly expensive, because in some areas financial arrangements must be made with the backup physician. For example, in California nurse-midwives work under the supervision of a physician. Should the parents sue for malpractice, it is the physician, not the midwife, who is responsible, unjust as this may be. Accordingly, the cost of midwifery is higher to cover the physician's malpractice insurance.

> ### Benefits of Midwifery Care
>
> The following are advantages associated with midwifery care. Bear in mind that the care midwives provide and their attitudes about childbirth vary from one practitioner to another.
>
> - Safe, personalized health care throughout the childbearing season
> - Non-interventive maternity care
> - Continuous emotional support through labor
> - Reduced chance of a cesarean section
> - Support of the mother and father's individual goals
> - Reduced cost in comparison to an obstetrician's care

Who Chooses Midwifery Care?

All mothers—low- and high-risk—can benefit from skilled, experienced midwifery care.

For home and childbearing center births, all responsible midwives screen mothers prenatally for complications. Most recommend that their clients also visit a physician to be checked out for conditions that may pose complications during pregnancy or labor. Women who have preeclampsia, kidney disease, heart disease, severe anemia, hypertension, diabetes, abnormal presentations, multiple gestations, placenta previa, pre- or postmature labor, and so on are usually referred to a physician.

In hospitals, unfortunately, midwives usually provide health care only to the low-risk mothers. There are exceptions. For instance, in New York City's North Central Bronx Hospital, where the population is predominantly high-risk, 100 percent of clients receive midwifery care, and 80 percent of births are midwife-attended. If there are medical complications, a physician may also give health care. But the midwife still remains actively involved.

The often-quoted studies about the safety of midwifery care in inner-city hospitals and rural areas have given many people the impression that midwives provide care for a primarily indigent population. This misconception leads some to assume that midwives provide second-class care. Both assumptions are myths.

Midwives provide care for mothers of all socioeconomic backgrounds. Surveys show that at least 25 percent of CNMs work in private practice offices with middle- to upper-income clients. Alice Bailes, CNM, of Birth Care and Women's Health in Alexandria, Virginia, for example, attends mothers of all backgrounds from the very upper-class to the indigent. Committed to helping women have safe births in the manner they choose, she has even attended a birth in a yurt (an eight-sided Tibetan sod house).

Though few midwives west of Tibet have a significant yurt birth population, most do provide care for a very wide clientele. Unfortunately, some people still have bizarre ideas about midwives. When they think of a midwife, the image of some back-country yahoo pops into mind. They don't realize that midwives are bona fide health professionals. Many parents and professionals don't know that many so-called lay midwives may be well-trained professionals with more skills than many physicians.

More mothers would opt for midwifery care if they learned about the safety of this care and what midwives offer. As one midwife puts it, "We have many uneducated consumers who come into nurse-midwifery by chance, not by seeking it. Once they are aware, they love it. We would have a larger clientele if people were more aware of what nurse-midwifery was."[2] Of course, this applies to direct-entry midwifery as well.

Choosing a Midwife

Both certified nurse-midwives and direct-entry midwives practice in every state in the United States. However, in states where direct-entry midwifery is not yet legal, midwives who will attend a home birth are not always easy to find. In fact, they remind me of the persecuted early Christians who lived in the catacombs. A mother from Indiana, a state where lay midwifery was illegal as of 1994, reveals, "After much searching, a CNM gave me the phone number of a lay midwife who would have been prosecuted had she been caught practicing."

When choosing a midwife, do the following:

◆ Ask about the midwife's background. Where was she trained? How many births has she attended? Midwives vary tremendously in their skill and experience. This is particularly true of those who don't have a license or certification. As Mary Hammond-Tooke of the Maternity Center in Bethesda, Maryland, puts it, "A lay midwife can include everyone from a woman who has watched a couple of births and thinks there is nothing to helping mothers through labor to someone who is highly trained, highly skilled, and very experienced." Though most midwives are highly skilled, some have little experience. Some even train on the job without any background or apprenticeship with more experienced practitioners. I can't overemphasize the need to select a skilled, experienced midwife.

◆ Find out about your midwife's backup and meet the backup physician. Everyone planning to give birth at home or in a birth center should have a backup physician and hospital in case a last-minute transfer is necessary.

◆ Find out the midwife's philosophy of birth and whether it agrees with yours. Midwives differ greatly in their approach. Some midwives do intervene unnecessarily; at the other extreme, a few midwives won't take any action to intervene even when necessary.

◆ Find out if your midwife will continue to provide maternity care and emotional support if you must be transferred from home or a childbearing center to the hospital. Whether or not the midwife remains with the mother throughout her hospital stay depends largely on her relationship with a backup physician and hospital. In some areas hospitals and backup physicians are not as supportive of midwives as they are in others, and your midwife may not be able to remain with you, through no fault of her own.

The Safety of Midwifery Care

Medical research has proven that for essentially normal, healthy pregnancies and labors, midwifery care is just as safe as physician care. Research shows that midwives working in collaboration with a physician are also safe health care providers for high-risk mothers. Midwifery care is safe under the following conditions:

◆ The midwife is well trained and experienced.

◆ The midwife works with a physician or has physician backup to handle complications during pregnancy and labor.

◆ The midwife who is not practicing in a hospital has adequate medical equipment and supplies, including oxygen and infant-resuscitation equipment.

◆ The midwife who attends childbearing center and home births has adequate backup at a nearby hospital.

Throughout the world medical studies have revealed midwifery care's impressive results. Research repeatedly proves that both direct-entry midwives and certified nurse-midwives have outstanding health statistics in home, childbearing center, and hospital settings.

Midwife-assisted births are associated with decreased infant mortality. As of 1994 the United States, with its large percentage of doctor-managed births, has one of the highest infant mortality rates on earth. Among the twenty-four largest industrialized nations, the United States ranks twenty-third in infant mortality. In Sweden, the country that ranks second lowest in infant mortality, nearly all mothers—even those with medical problems requiring the help of a physician—receive midwifery care.[3]

In the Netherlands, a country with one of the world's lowest infant mortality rates, midwives care for nearly all pregnant and laboring women. The Dutch government, which pays for medical services for 70 percent of the population, will not pay for a physician to attend childbirth unless the mother has a medical complication.

In other countries with low infant mortality rates, including Finland, Denmark, Norway, and Switzerland, midwives attend most births. Of course, other factors, such as good nutrition, may be partly responsible for the low rates. However, we should not underestimate the role midwifery plays in the care of the healthy mother and child.

Midwifery care for essentially healthy mothers giving birth at home or in childbearing centers is as safe, if not safer, than obstetrician care in the hospital. Some physicians claim that midwifery care, particularly at home, is fraught with more medical problems and deaths than physician care in the hospital. Studies show the very opposite! People who claim physician-attended hospital birth is safer usually base their comparison on unskilled midwifery care (which isn't midwifery care at all) and unsupervised birth at home. As medical statistician David Stewart points out, "Raw data for 'out-of-hospital births' are always worse than for hospitals. This is because such data usually include accidents on the way to the hospital, miscarriages at home, economically mandated home births, and even homicide (pregnant teenagers giving birth unattended and leaving their babies to die of exposure)."[4]

Two associate professors of sociology at Arizona State University, Deborah Sullivan and Rose Weitz, conducted a fascinating study. They wondered why in the world any mother would give birth at home with a lay midwife when she could have an obstetrician help her in a top hospital. The results of their study were nothing less than mind-boggling. They reviewed 3,257 out-of-hospital births occurring from 1978 to 1985. Arizona-licensed midwives who carried no health care degrees managed the births. The perinatal mortality rate was 2.2 per thousand and the neonatal mortality rate was 1.1 per thousand.[5] (The perinatal mortality rate refers to the combined total of fetal deaths occurring on or after twenty-eight weeks of gestation and within the first twenty-eight days of life outside the uterus. Neonatal mortality is the statistical rate of infant death during the first twenty-eight days after birth.) By comparison, the United States infant mortality rate for 1987 was 10.5 per thousand.[6] The sociologists published this eye-opening study in their book *Labor Pains*, which includes hundreds of medical references supporting the safety of midwifery care. This book alone is enough to convince any open-minded reader of the safety of midwifery care and the relative danger of conventional physician-managed maternity care.

But it is by no means an isolated study. Research in Mississippi showed that the infant mortality rates for the state were almost cut in half (from thirty-eight to twenty per thousand) two years after certified nurse-midwives began providing primary care to pregnant women.

The certified nurse-midwives of the Maternity Center in Bethesda, Maryland, have been attending the births of twenty to twenty-five carefully selected mothers monthly. They attended exclusively home births from 1975 to 1982 and then began attending childbearing center births. Today about three-quarters of the births take place in the center and about a quarter occur at home. "Among all of the out-of-hospital births," says Mary Hammond-Tooke, CNM, of the Maternity Center, "there have been no maternal deaths and we have never had a baby die because of the planned place of birth." The perinatal deaths that did occur resulted from such unavoidable problems as severe congenital abnormalities that would have had the same outcome in the hospital as well.

A fascinating community supporting natural childbirth and midwifery is The Farm in Summertown, Tennessee. The Farm is a spiritual and agricultural community where midwives attend all births. Though all the midwives have experience and clinical skills, *none has formal medical training.* The midwives' statistics probably remain unmatched by any hospital in the world. Out of one thousand mothers who gave birth at The Farm between 1970 and 1979, the perinatal mortality rate was fifteen (including mothers who required transfer to the hospital). By comparison, the rate for Tennessee during this time was twenty per thousand and the rate for the United States was double that of The Farm's—thirty per thousand. Only 4 percent of the mothers at The Farm transferred to the hospital, and the cesarean section rate was 1.5 percent.[7]

Experienced, skilled midwives have health statistics superior to the national average even when working with high-risk clients in both home and hospital settings. Midwives usually take care of low-risk clients, referring those at high risk of pregnancy or labor complications to obstetricians. In light of this, it isn't surprising that midwives might have better health statistics. However, many medical studies show midwifery care has also had a dramatic impact on improving the health of high-risk mothers and babies. In all settings midwives spell a reduction in low birth weight, prematurity, and neonatal mortality.

The population of North Central Bronx Hospital is mostly black and Hispanic mothers, many of whom are at high risk of complications, yet medical intervention is minimal. Membranes are not artificially ruptured, pain-relief medication or regional anesthesia is administered in fewer than 30 percent of births, and Pitocin is used to augment labor in only 3 percent of cases. Eighty-five percent of mothers give birth in a semisitting position without stirrups, and forceps are used in fewer than 3 percent of births. The prevailing philosophy of the midwives at this hospital includes providing emotional support to all women. Mothers have freedom to eat, drink, and walk around during labor.

What are the results of this maternity care? According to medical statistician Dr. David Stewart, "With a population of mothers at considerably higher than average risk, the midwives of North Central Bronx have achieved better maternal and infant outcomes than the rest of New York City, the State of New York in general, and the United States as a whole. There isn't a single hospital in the entire country with populations of similar risk run by doctors with results as good as this one run by midwives."[8]

A revealing study done in Madera County, California, also makes a dramatic case for midwifery. The study compares the health statistics of obstetricians, family physicians, and nurse midwives. The results are dramatic. The mothers at Madera County Hospital are mostly poor agricultural workers at high risk for complications. In 1959, when family physicians staffed the hospital, the neonatal mortality rate was a high 23.9 per thousand births. From 1960 to 1963 the state of California brought nurse-midwives to the hospital. What occurred? The neonatal mortality rate plummeted to 10.3 per thousand. Despite the high-risk population, this statistic was better than the average for the entire state!

When obstetricians replaced midwives in 1964, one might have expected these highly trained specialists to produce even greater improvement. But what happened would be almost un-believable if it were not recorded in black and white. The neonatal mortality rate more than tripled to 32.1 per thousand.[9] The results of this study are so astounding that one might think it an isolated case, yet differences between midwifery and obstetrical care have produced similar striking health statistics throughout the world.

The well-known Frontier Nursing Service (FNS) is a legend of the impressively good health statistics of midwifery care for high-risk women. Mary Breckenridge founded FNS in 1925. She brought British-trained nurse-midwives to Kentucky to provide maternity care for people living in a rural area. The Metropolitan Life

Insurance Company tabulated their statistics. Between 1925 and 1951 Frontier Nursing Service midwives provided maternity care for 8,596 women. Of these, 6,533 gave birth at home, primarily in primitive conditions. The maternal death rate was 1.2 per thousand, quite high by today's standards. Yet it was one-third the maternal mortality rate for the United States as a whole then, which was 3.4 per thousand. The service's neonatal mortality rate for the early 1950s was less than the average for Kentucky and the United States as a whole.

In 1985 the Institute of Medicine published a comprehensive report about ways to prevent low birth weight, a major cause of neonatal morbidity, or illness. The report concluded that certified nurse-midwives were particularly effective in managing the care of women who were at high risk because of social and economic factors. The institute suggested probable reasons for the superior results midwives achieve with high-risk clients: Midwives don't set themselves up as "authority figures" when relating to their patients. They emphasize education, emotional support, and client satisfaction. As a result, women are more likely to keep prenatal care appointments with nurse-midwives than with physicians. The Institute of Medicine also proposed increasing midwives' hospital privileges.

Why Are Midwifery Statistics So Impressive?

Why do skilled, experienced midwives have such outstanding health statistics? How can midwives often boast of better health statistics than obstetricians? There is no single answer.

One important reason, however, is that most midwives do not routinely use such medical intervention as electronic fetal monitoring. They reserve obstetrical procedures for those who need them. We cannot overemphasize the dire result of unnecessary medical intervention. Researcher Dr. Lewis Mehl compared a matched population of 2,092 home and hospital birth mothers in the states of Wisconsin and California. Lay midwives attended 31 percent of the home births, nurse-midwives attended 2 percent, and family physicians attended 67 percent. Among hospital births, obstetricians attended 75 percent and family physicians attended 25 percent. The fetal distress rate was *six times* higher in the hospital group. Three times as many maternal hemorrhages occurred. Three times the number of babies needed resuscitation. Four times as many babies got neonatal infections. Physicians caused thirty permanent birth injuries (primarily by using forceps).[10]

Another reason for midwives' success is that many midwives understand the emotional and the physical needs of the laboring woman. As a result, the midwife often has something I call an *opening presence*. Her personality and nurturing care encourage the mother to surrender to labor, facilitating its progress.

Furthermore, most midwives remain with the mother throughout labor. Studies have shown that continuous emotional support can reduce the pain, the length, and the incidence of complications in labor.

Finally, in my opinion, the most important factor in the midwife's superior health care statistics is her conscious or unconscious understanding of the laboring mind response (see chapter 2). Bear in mind that the emotions influence labor. Meeting the laboring woman's emotional needs is as important as meeting her physical needs.

Physician Backup and Hospital Privileges

All midwives should have a collaborative relationship with physicians for consultation and referral. This safety net is essential for maternal-infant health. A physician should be readily available should complications require a doctor's care. However, many midwives, particularly direct-entry midwives, cannot find a physician willing to back them up. In the words of one physician who supports midwifery care, "The focus should be on the patient, not the practitioner. When we deny backup to midwives, we are telling the patient she doesn't have the right to the medical care she chooses. And we are denying her the health care to which every person is entitled."

Professor Helen Varney of the maternal-newborn program at Yale University argues that CNMs should be able to admit clients to the hospital, practice the full scope of midwifery within the hospital, and discharge clients. CNMs who practice in childbearing centers or homes also need full hospital privileges so that they can provide continuity of care to women who require a transfer.

However, this hardly means physicians should *control* midwives. Nearly all midwives, just like all physicians, justifiably feel they should regulate their own profession. I believe the midwife-physician relationship should be a mutual one of equals, not one in which the physician has supervisory powers. Ideally, the midwife should function autonomously, creating his or her own rules and protocol. Allowing physicians to control the practice and privileges of midwives is an absurdity that gives one profession the power to restrain another profession, not unlike organized crime. It is like allowing Burger King to have the final say when and where McDonald's will be permitted to sell hamburgers!

Laws Governing Midwives

Certified nurse-midwives are licensed to practice in all fifty states of the United States. In some states, however, only a handful of hospitals give privileges to CNMs. In other states, such as California, New York, and Florida, many certified nurse-midwives work in hospitals. Every year more hospitals open their doors to midwives.

Direct-entry midwives are governed by regulations that vary dramatically from state to state within the United States.

In a few states, lay midwives are licensed, registered, or certified. However, what they can do varies from one state to another. For example, in New Hampshire, lay midwives are certified to offer prenatal care, assistance during labor, and postpartum care. The New Hampshire Department of Health and Human Services regulates their practice. To become certified, midwives must meet state requirements for training and for clinical and home birth experience and pass an exam. Once certified, they may practice in both home and freestanding birth centers. Meanwhile, lay midwives who are not certified can also practice legally.

In some states no laws govern direct-entry midwives. The midwives of these states are self-regulating. For example, in Vermont, where direct-entry midwives call themselves "independent midwives," midwifery is neither legal nor illegal. There is no state certification or licensing board. However, midwife Laurie Foster, who practices in both Vermont and New Hampshire, points out that , "the Vermont Midwives Alliance has its own standards of protocol, which are quite similar to the standards for the state of New Hampshire."

In Arizona, direct-entry midwives call themselves "licensed midwives." The Arizona Department of Health Services licenses the midwife after she has completed an approved course of instruction and passed state-administered exams. She can then provide care for essentially normal women and their newborns. Her practice embraces prenatal care, help in home and childbearing center birth, and postpartum care. In states where lay midwifery is still illegal, midwives who provide much-needed maternity care do so at risk of fines and even imprisonment.

In most states direct-entry midwives attend only home births. In a few locations they can also provide care in childbearing centers. Consider the Netherlands and Denmark, by contrast. There the direct-entry midwife provides maternity care wherever birth takes place. It was only in 1990 that direct-entry midwives in the United States began applying for hospital privileges.

Laws regulating midwifery practice are changing rapidly throughout the United States. Some of these laws desperately need change. For example, not long ago in Massachusetts, a state infamous for peculiar laws, it was illegal for a certified nurse-midwife to attend a home birth but legal for another professional— say, for example, a plumber—to do so. The law has since changed. In other states midwives who have better health statistics than physicians have been fined and even imprisoned for practicing.

Laws legalizing lay midwifery can be both good and bad for midwives and clients. Legislation protects the consumer by establishing standards of competency. But it can also tie the midwife's hands by prohibiting the use of drugs, requiring collaboration and backup by physicians, and so on.

As of 1994, the ACNM is the only nationally recognized accrediting organization for midwives in the United States. All nationally certified midwives are certified nurse-midwives. However, midwives are actively working toward getting official recognition for direct-entry midwives. I hope the Dutch model of midwifery will one day be adopted in the United States and elsewhere.

Some direct-entry midwives resist this change. Understandably, they don't want to risk losing their autonomy. Nor do they want to be under the supervision of physicians, particularly when physicians have exercised restraint of trade, keeping them from practicing. Nevertheless, to ensure that every licensed direct-entry midwife has a minimum level of education and practical experience in obstetrics, most midwives agree we should adopt a single standard of professional midwifery in the United States.

With little doubt midwives, like physicians, will soon be self-regulating in every state, with the full privileges their profession requires.

Opposition to Midwives

Some physicians respect midwifery services, while others disagree with the very idea of midwifery. Certified nurse-midwife Elizabeth Clifton, who runs a birthing center in Missouri, says of her area, "The medical profession considers midwives of any stripe—whether they be lay midwives, certified nurse midwives, or have a Ph.D. behind their name—absolute anathema." Though this statement is hardly true nationwide, there are still thousands of hospitals across the country where CNMs cannot practice.

In the words of Ernest L. Boyer, president of the Carnegie Foundation for the Advancement of Teaching, "Midwives have been subjected to a relentless campaign of innuendo and invective, a maliciously destructive crusade that not only challenged their professional competence, but debased their character as well."[11]

The opposition to midwifery—ranging from prejudice based on ignorance to outright persecution—is not unlike the response physicians made to Ignaz Philipp Semmelweiss, the first physician to prove the cause of puerperal fever. When Dr. Semmelweiss, a Viennese physician, observed that the mortality rate of mothers in the medical students' ward was 437 percent greater than the rate in the midwives' ward, he concluded that doctors were transmitting the disease. He also discovered the cure: antiseptic hand washing. Doctors ridiculed him for this, refusing to believe what the statistics clearly showed. One respected physician even argued that physicians were gentlemen whose hands were clean.[12] For that matter, many have justifiably likened the persecution of midwives under the name of unfair laws to the witch-hunts of the Middle Ages.

Witch-hunting and the epidemic of puerperal fever are things of the past, but ignorance remains. Many doctors still refuse to pay attention to the statistics showing midwifery care is as safe as—if not safer than—physician care. Like the doctors in the nineteenth century, they are still ridiculing those who show us how to reduce infant and maternal disease. Many physicians fear that midwives lack both education and high standards of practice. While it is true that many direct-entry midwives have no certification board or committee of medical professionals, and a few lack skills and experience, most midwives offer very high standards of maternity care. Other physicians hold the genuine belief that obstetricians provide safer care for mothers and babies. Despite information to the contrary published in their own journals, many obstetricians (and parents) so strongly believe that mothers need technological intervention to give birth safely that facts don't seem to persuade them otherwise. `

Another reason for the prejudice may be that midwives and physicians are essentially competing for the same middle- to upper-class clients. As one physician puts it, "Those physicians who see CNMs as a threat to the pocketbook take refuge behind all kinds of philosophical and medical baloney." Midwives can offer equal if not superior health care at less cost than obstetricians. The motive behind some physicians' opposition may simply be to eliminate competition. Medical statistician David Stewart observes that the "dramatic disappearance of a centuries-old profession, almost to extinction, was no accident."[13]

Meanwhile, opposition between midwives and physicians is not entirely one-sided. A few midwives have been equally hostile toward the medical profession. A handful of vocal midwives seem to be waging an angry campaign against what they perceive as the male-dominated medical establishment, and a small number oppose medical care of any kind. For example, one midwife told me she refused to learn suturing because she might be tempted to use the technique! Opposition to conventional medical care is waxing in popularity as more people become disgusted with medicine's disease-oriented view. However, a midwife who refuses to learn lifesaving medical techniques is as ignorant as the physician who does not recognize other forms of treatment, from acupuncture to chiropractic care. Fortunately for mothers, these midwives represent a tiny minority.

Hostility accomplishes nothing. Safe maternity care of the

mother's choice in the setting she prefers will exist only if all childbirth professionals—midwives, physicians, childbirth educators, and nurses, male and female—accept, respect, and support one another's work.

Looking Ahead

The increasing popularity of the midwife—including physicians and naturopaths who practice like midwives—is perhaps the single greatest stride toward safer, rewarding births in the United States and Canada in the twentieth century.

If current trends in midwifery continue, midwives will grow in numbers and become far more popular than they are today. The outdated hospitals that now deny nurse-midwives privileges will either open their doors to this increasingly popular childbirth professional or succumb to competitors. I believe we will also soon welcome a new professional to the established system of medical care: the number of direct-entry midwives will grow as well. They will become legitimate, their practice recognized, and their work respected throughout the world.

Perhaps midwifery will become the standard of maternity care. As direct-entry midwife Joan Remington asserts, "There is no doubt we will have a significant impact on lowering perinatal mortality, as every study in the United States and overseas has proven over and over."

Most important, whoever provides health care—physician or midwife—will place greater emphasis on the emotional needs of the family throughout the childbearing drama. This change, in turn, will spell more positive birth experiences for the entire family. The midwife will again become what she has always been since the dawn of history: a central figure in maternal-child health care.

And you and your baby will benefit.

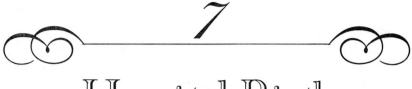

Hospital Birth Choices

Bev, a mother of two, gave birth in a hospital whose staff was wholly committed to supporting her birth plans. "The birthing room," she recalls, "was filled with warmth, smiles, and wonder. My husband, Greg, and I had the kind of childbirth experience we wanted: family-oriented, no routine electronic monitoring, no episiotomy—soft lights and a warm, inviting room with regular old beds. The staff respected our wishes and welcomed our four-year-old son Joshua to share in the joy and the miracle of birth.

"My labor went quickly. Contractions were intense but controllable with no special breathing needed. Second stage lasted only fifteen minutes. As the baby was born, Joshua sat on my midwife's lap at the edge of the bed, wide-eyed. The physician dimmed the lights. I could feel myself opening, stretching wider and wider with an intense burning feeling. Short quick breaths helped me relax, and my body eased the baby out. The beautiful baby I longed to greet was placed on my belly. Together our family welcomed seven-pound, twelve-ounce, twenty-one-inch Heather Elizabeth into a sensitive, gentle, intimate world."

Hospital birth can be a wonderful, rewarding event, a memory forever cherished. Or it can be a nightmare. One can no more make blanket statements about giving birth in hospitals than one can make generalizations about eating in restaurants. Some give you fond memories. Others make you wish you had never walked in the door. You must assess each hospital individually.

Fortunately, a more humanized maternity care is evolving in hospitals. Many are remodeling the once-clinical and impersonal settings called labor and delivery rooms to seem more homelike.

More important, the philosophy of maternity care in many hospitals is being revolutionized.

"It's exciting!" exclaims the birthing unit nurse manager of a hospital whose staff recently adopted a new approach to maternity care where the family's needs come before policy. "I've been working here twenty years. For the first time we're finally almost to the point where laboring women—I should say, families—are giving birth the way they should."

Following are some of the many factors that are contributing to the changes taking place in hospitals:

- The increasing popularity of home and childbearing center birth is forcing change. In some California suburbs, 10 percent of mothers gave birth at home during the mid-1970s. In response, the number of birth rooms in hospitals increased from 3 in 1975 to 120 in 1982. This development of more humanized hospital birth is an attempt to mimic home birth.[1]

- The women's movement, with its emphasis on women's taking control of their own bodies and health care, is inspiring change.

- Consumer-oriented childbirth education classes have made more parents aware of the birth options and the disadvantages and risks involved in medical interventions and procedures.

- Consumer pressure for a more humanized birth experience is inspiring hospitals to make changes. The most significant factor is you, the health care consumer. You shape your own birth. As more expectant parents realize this—instead of blaming doctors, hospitals, and insurance companies—change will take place in the consumer's favor.

- Many childbirth professionals, particularly nurses, who are often the most instrumental in triggering change, are becoming increasingly aware of the laboring mind response. They are beginning to realize that satisfying the emotional dimensions of the birth experience—the need for peace, privacy, a positive emotional climate, a supportive birth partner—can contribute to better maternal-infant health.

The Safety of Hospital Birth

Most American parents and physicians take the safety of hospital birth for granted. The vast majority assume that the hospital is the safest birth environment. This is a cultural belief, not a scientific fact. The Dutch, unlike Americans and Canadians, do not hold this view. And the Dutch have one of the world's lowest infant mortality rates. Half the population gives birth at home.

Many are surprised to learn that there is not one medical study proving hospital birth to be safer than planned home or childbearing center birth for the essentially normal mother. (See chapter 9 for studies comparing the safety of hospital births versus home births.) Proponents of hospital birth point out that unforeseen complications are better handled in the hospital setting than elsewhere.

Though hospital birth *is* safe for most mothers, medical studies have shown that there is an increased risk of maternal and infant morbidity (illness) in the hospital as compared to home. The risk of infection to mother and baby is greater in the hospital (where there are more disease-causing organisms) than at home. In fact, the first U.S. rooming-in program, established in the 1940s at Duke University in North Carolina, was created not to promote maternal-infant attachment but to avoid severe nursery epidemics of infant diarrhea.

Varying with the hospital, the mother and baby are also at higher risk of iatrogenic (doctor-caused) complications. These include such problems as fetal distress caused by overuse of oxytocic drugs to stimulate labor or by pain-relief medication, infections from too many vaginal exams, unnecessary surgical birth, and the baby blues.

The baby blues (described in chapter 4) are significantly more common following hospital than home or childbearing center birth. In a British study pediatrician Aidan MacFarlane showed that 68 percent of hospital birth mothers experienced baby blues, compared to 16 percent of home birth mothers.

Giving birth in a hospital with an emotionally positive climate where maternity care is individualized can dramatically reduce all these risks.

Who Gives Birth in the Hospital?

The overwhelming majority of American mothers give birth in hospitals. Most who choose the hospital do so because they feel safest in that setting. The mothers who benefit most from in-hospital birth include:

- Mothers who have previously existing medical complications or who are considered at high risk for having problems during childbearing
- Mothers who feel more comfortable and safer in the hospital for any reason
- Mothers who cannot find a competent home birth practitioner or childbearing center in their area

The Pros and Cons of Hospital Birth

The advantages of hospital birth are as follows:

- The hospital is the safest environment for the mother at risk of medical complications during labor. Women with such medical problems as heart disease, diabetes, or complications like preeclampsia (a pregnancy disease characterized by high blood pressure, protein in the urine, and excessive swelling) are safest in the hospital where medical intervention is immediately available. For instance, an emergency cesarean delivery can be performed immediately.
- Many women feel safest and most comfortable in the hospital. Many feel secure giving birth in a homelike setting in the hospital with the knowledge that the latest technological equipment and expert care are just a step away.
- Immediate pediatric attention is available should the baby have medical problems. Intensive care and a pediatrician or neonatologist are available twenty-four hours a day in a tertiary or level III facility—that is, a hospital well equipped to handle major problems. In most hospitals, however, a baby requiring intensive care often must be transferred to another facility with an intensive care center.

Despite the benefits, hospital birth carries some risks and disadvantages. I have yet to meet the mother who has experienced both a rewarding hospital and joyful home birth and prefers the former. "Hospital birth—despite how beautiful the environment and how supportive the staff—can never quite match home birth for peace and comfort," says Dr. Howard Marchbanks, an obstetrician who attends births in homes, childbearing centers, and hospitals in Orange County, California.

Few hospitals have the positive emotional climate of childbearing centers. As Eunice Ernst of the National Association of Childbearing Centers puts it, "The contemporary hospital setting is a quantum leap away from the freestanding birth center. It is an attempt to accommodate the acute care setting to women who are not sick." This situation is changing, however, as hospitals develop their own birth centers.

Disadvantages of hospital birth vary from one institution to another. They include the following:

- The risk of iatrogenic complications and infection to mother and baby is greater in a hospital birth than in a home or childbearing center birth.

- The mother is at a significantly higher risk of having an unnecessary cesarean section, especially in a hospital with a high cesarean rate. Though some cesareans save the life of mother or baby, the vast majority are avoidable. It is far more difficult to avoid unnecessary surgery in a hospital with a 25 to 30 percent cesarean rate than it is in a childbearing center with only a 3 to 4 percent rate. (This rate refers to mothers transferred to the hospital for cesareans that are usually necessary. Again, childbearing centers screen for low-risk pregnancies, so their rate is lower.)

- The father is often less actively involved in the childbearing process in the hospital than he is in the childbearing center or at home.

- The parents are not on home ground and don't have the same control as they do at home.

- Hospitals are associated with illness. Birth is a normal, natural event, not an illness.

- Most hospitals are not restful. Some think getting rest is an advantage of hospital birth because they can remain in the hospital longer than in some birth centers if they prefer. This is a misconception. The quality of rest one gets in a hospital is often poor. Few hospitals provide truly restful environments. As one nurse puts it, "If rest is your goal, it would be better to turn to the experts in the field, namely, the hotel and resort industry."

Settings for Hospital Birth

A wide range of settings are available in today's hospitals for labor, birth, and the early postpartum period. Being acquainted with these will help you make the best choice of maternity hospital in your area. Many conventional hospital labor and delivery units are not really conducive to normal labor. They are sterile, clinical environments, polluted by the jarring noise of loudspeakers, where the mother is not as comfortable as she would be in a more homelike setting. In addition, the narrow beds common in most hospitals do not allow the mother freedom of movement or have room for the father to be with his mate, holding, caressing, and supporting her.

THE LABOR AND DELIVERY ROOM

In the traditional hospital birth of the 1970s and 1980s, the mother labored in a labor room, usually a typical hospital room designed for one or two persons. Then, close to the time of giving birth, she was moved to a separate, sterile delivery room. After giving birth, she was moved to a third room, called a recovery room. Then anytime from minutes to hours afterward, she moved to yet a fourth room in a postpartum unit. In conventional hospital delivery, the newborn was also typically transferred to no fewer than four rooms—from the delivery room to a transitional nursery, then to a newborn nursery, then to the mother's room for feeding (if the mother did not have twenty-four-hour rooming-in), and back again to the nursery.

Moving women and babies about from room to room during childbearing is one of America's most peculiar customs. Constant transfer is traumatic for the mother, who during labor is vulnerable and sensitive; upsetting for the father, who often must change into

Hospital Birth Settings

The following can be comfortable settings conducive to a safe, positive labor, delivery, and early postpartum period. Bear in mind that setting alone does not create a rewarding birth. These settings are conducive to a positive birth only in hospitals with flexible policies, supportive health care providers, and a nursing staff who view the mother as essentially healthy.

◆ *Birthing room.* A room where the mother labors, gives birth, and usually remains for the first postpartum hour or so. Birthing rooms are usually designed only for low-risk mothers. This term is sometimes used interchangeably with LDR, LDRP, and ABC.

◆ *Labor, delivery, recovery room* (LDR). A room in which the mother (usually regardless of risk status) labors, gives birth, and spends the first hour or so after birth.

◆ *Labor, delivery, recovery, postpartum room* (LDRP). A room in which the mother (usually regardless of risk status) labors, gives birth, and remains during the postpartum period throughout her hospital stay.

◆ *Alternative birth center (ABC), also called family birth center* (FBC) or *twenty-four-hour suite.* A homelike facility for labor and birth, consisting of a suite of rooms where the childbearing family remains from admission to discharge.

scrub clothes in a rush; and a shock to the newborn. Further, it is a waste of hospital space and personnel hours. While a delivery room is a good setting for operative obstetrics because it is an operating room, it is about as suitable for beginning a family as a car wash is for celebrating a honeymoon.

This multitransfer style of maternity care was modeled on the surgical system. Not long ago it was the rule in all maternity hospitals. Though a few hospitals still maintain the practice, it has fortunately become largely a thing of history as more health professionals realize that it serves no useful purpose and is a waste of time and money.

Types of Hospitals

When choosing a hospital it's important to know the three basic types. These classifications are determined by the availability of emergency medical care.

- A *Level I facility* or *primary care center* provides health care to low-risk clients. Its services include the identification of high-risk pregnancies, health care during unanticipated obstetric or newborn emergencies, and care of normal newborns. Level I facilities are frequently in sparsely populated areas. Often there is no anesthesiologist in the birth unit, and it may take thirty minutes or more to set up for a cesarean section.

- A *Level II facility* or secondary care center offers care to the majority of clients and is able to provide care in about 90 percent of maternal or neonatal complications, as well as low-risk care. It usually takes only five to ten minutes to set up for an emergency cesarean in such a facility.

- A *Level III facility* or *tertiary care center* provides care for high-risk clients who require the most sophisticated type of medical and technical intervention. Full-time specialists and the most modern equipment are available around the clock, and emergency cesareans can be done immediately. The tertiary care center is best for certain life-threatening emergencies, neonatal surgery, very premature labors, and other medical complications. The atmosphere is usually highly clinical and therefore not ideal for normal birth.

CONTEMPORARY HOSPITAL FACILITIES

Contemporary maternity facilities allow mother and baby to remain in the same room or, at most, two rooms throughout their hospital stay. When you think about it, there is really nothing new about this idea. Women have been laboring, giving birth, and remaining with their babies in the same room for as long as they've lived in homes. Still, for hospitals the idea was revolutionary and represented an entirely new idea in maternity care.

According to the American Hospital Association, as of 1987 nearly 80 percent of American hospitals had birthing rooms or other similar rooms, though these hospitals did not all use the single room units regularly. The rooms vary as much as hotel rooms in appearance. Some are little different from ordinary labor rooms, with a narrow bed and a nearby chair; others are beautifully furnished. Many have a single or double bed, pictures, wallpaper, comfortable chairs, and a private shower or bath.[2]

Medical equipment and sterile instrument supplies are usually out of sight. For example, in the Family Birthing Center of Manchester Memorial Hospital in Connecticut all medical equipment is in the hallways, close by but out of the parents' view. In many other birthing rooms I have visited, the medical supplies are in a closet that also contains emergency equipment for an infant requiring pediatric attention.

Some hospital settings, such as the Birth Place at St. Mary's Hospital in Minneapolis, have double beds. Unfortunately, most hospital maternity rooms have very narrow beds. This inhibits the mother from changing position as she pleases and leaves little or no room for the father. As far as I'm concerned, the beds in all birthing rooms should be double or queen-sized to allow both parents plenty of room.

The lights are usually dimmed as the parents desire. Most laboring women prefer a dimly lit room. Lighting should also be subdued after the baby is born, as bright light hurts the sensitive newborn's eyes and will cause her to squint. In a dimly lit room, the infant will open her eyes and gaze at her parents' faces.

An ordinary labor room can be used for both labor and birth if the parents wish and the hospital permits. The labor room is used both for labor and birth in some hospitals that have not remodeled to create single-room maternity care. If birthing rooms, LDRs, or LDRPs are not yet available in your area, you may be able to arrange a labor room birth in your local hospital with your health care provider's approval even if it is not standard hospital practice.

More important than the physical setup is the philosophy behind the maternity care. "Look beyond the decorated birthing rooms," advises Dr. Celeste Phillips, former clinical obstetrical specialist for the Surgeon General's Office and founder of Phillips and Fenwick, a firm helping hospitals create family-centered maternity care programs. "What is the philosophy behind those rooms? What does the staff believe about childbirth? It's the people who create good maternity care, the people and what they believe." As Susan Driesel of the Medical Center in Tulsa, Oklahoma, puts it, "Many hospitals spend much time and money creating the physical environment but don't consider the philosophy behind that environment."

Obstetrician Richard Stewart describes the philosophy behind the homelike Douglasville Birthing Center he created: "We view birth as a social, emotional, and psychological event as well as a medical event. Therefore, the attitude of calm, quiet, and peace leads to much less necessary medical intervention. Medical intervention in hospitals is a pyramid phenomenon. As we are all aware, one intervention leads to another. The mother who receives Pitocin often needs pain-relief medication. The medication often leads to more Pitocin. This can lead to an epidural that can lead to forceps delivery and an episiotomy. There are dozens of examples of the way this works. However, the initial intervention is often unnecessary if the mother is not tense or afraid, has someone she knows supporting her throughout labor, and is able to labor in a peaceful, homelike environment surrounded by family and friends."

A new philosophy of hospital maternity care is evolving, in many ways similar to the home birth philosophy. "Most American nurses and health professionals used to view laboring women as sick patients," says Colleen Gerlach, head nurse of the Birthplace at Riverside Medical Center in Minneapolis. "Many still do. However, now...we view childbirth as a function of being well. The nurses and the health care providers—midwives, family practitioners, and obstetricians—support the family versus deliver the mother. Rather than think of the laboring mother as ill, we look at her as probably the healthiest she's ever going to be in her life, going through the normal process of childbearing."

The staff at the Family Maternity Center at Holy Family Hospital in Spokane, Washington, view expectant mothers as partners in their care. The health care varies according to a plan that parents design with their physician. The parents actively participate in all decisions about labor and childbirth. Fathers are always welcome to participate in the birth, including being present at emergency cesareans where general anesthesia is used. The cesarean delivery rate is 6.8 percent, less than one-third the national average. Nurses either make home visits or follow-up telephone calls (at the parents' choice) during the early postpartum period. As Frances S. Waryas, RN, of patient care services, and Matthew B. Luebbers, administrator, so eloquently sum up: "Perhaps the key to the center's success is the belief held by staff members that childbirth is not a technical exercise but rather a celebration of life. This philosophy of care is practiced daily."[3]

BIRTHING ROOMS

In many states the birthing room is a room providing family-centered care in a homelike environment for low-risk mothers throughout the labor, delivery, and immediate postpartum recovery period. However, some hospitals use the terms *birthing room, LDR,* and *LDRP* interchangeably.

The first birthing room in the United States opened in 1969 at Manchester Memorial Hospital in Manchester, Connecticut, under the direction of pioneer obstetrician Dr. Philip Sumner. This hospital has recently remodeled and opened the Family Birthing Center, with six birthing rooms. All mothers give birth in these rooms whether their risk is high or low. The only other rooms for birth are two cesarean rooms used solely for surgical delivery.

The care, policies, and atmosphere in birthing rooms vary tremendously from one institution to another. Some birthing rooms are tranquil, pleasant settings where individualized maternity care, flexible policies, and unrestricted contact with the baby after birth are the rule. Others embrace routine medical procedures and rigid policies.

In many hospitals, birthing rooms are little more than an advertising ploy to get people in the door. For example, in one of the most horrendous hospitals I've ever seen, where I was helping a woman through labor, there was no difference I could see in either policies or furnishings between birthing rooms and labor rooms.

When the mother and I arrived at the hospital, a nurse led us through a basement to what she called a "labor pod."

"What's a pod?" I asked.

"This is it," she said, indicating the entire labor and delivery area.

She then took us to a windowless, concrete cell with a narrow bed, a bed table with an electronic fetal monitor on top and a drawer stuffed with medical equipment, and a chair.

"Where are the birthing rooms?" I asked, still unsure what a pod was.

"These are the birthing rooms!"

I was astounded that such a horrible birth environment could exist. Even the back seat of a taxicab would have been more comfortable. Throughout the mother's labor, loudspeakers blared uninterrupted interruptions, the nurses made us feel as welcome as a swarm of mosquitoes, and the policies were as inflexible as those of a prison camp.

Don't depend on hospital literature for information on birthing rooms. Birthing rooms and other contemporary settings frequently offer only the illusion of a rewarding birth. Sociologist Raymond DeVries, who has studied hospital birth alternatives, has pointed out how birthing rooms and similar settings within the hospital have mimicked the physical environment of home while maintaining an interventive approach toward maternity care, medical control, and inflexible policies. His study of birth settings in the state of Washington revealed no difference in labor options between hospitals with and without birthing rooms. Major obstetrical interventions, including cesarean section and forceps delivery, have increased in some hospitals with birthing rooms.[4]

Visit the birthing rooms and talk with the staff. For example, before making a final choice, Evelyn, a mother of two in central Vermont, visited several facilities. "The two larger hospitals in my area had birthing rooms," she recalls. "However, the atmosphere was clinical and sterile. Policies unnecessarily restricted the mother's movements and the father's involvement. After talking with friends, we chose a small hospital with birthing rooms where the staff treat laboring women as people first, patients second."

The requirements for using the birthing room vary widely from one hospital to another. In some states regulations specify that birthing rooms are only for low-risk mothers. If such medical problems as fetal distress or elevated maternal temperature arise, the laboring woman transfers to a room more fully equipped for handling complications. A mother may also transfer because of her requests for medication, which is not available in many birthing rooms. If you want regional anesthesia—an epidural, for example—the regulations of some states require that you transfer to another room.

Some hospitals place absurd requirements on mothers, preventing many perfectly healthy women from using the birthing room. Often mothers under or over a certain age or those planning a vaginal birth after a previous cesarean are excluded. Also, some hospitals require the mother and father to take special birthing room classes before permitting them to use the room.

Dr. Celeste Phillips warns parents to beware of hospitals that place these kinds of restrictions on birth. Such policies suggest a staff so far from supportive that the mother jeopardizes her birth experience as soon as she walks through the door.

LDRs and LDRPs

Labor, deliver, recovery rooms (LDRs) and labor, delivery, recovery, postpartum rooms (LDRPs) are becoming the most popular options in maternity care. These units combine the homelike setting of the birthing room with the medical equipment and emergency support of a delivery room. In most hospitals LDRs accommodate both low- and high-risk labors. (Birthing rooms are generally limited to low-risk labors.) LDRs and LDRPs are usually larger as well as more fully equipped than birthing rooms.

LDR rooms are for labor, birth, and the first hour or so after birth, after which the mother moves to a postpartum area.

LDRP rooms are for the entire childbearing process, including care for the mother through labor, birth, and the early postpartum period, and also newborn care. Both LDRs and LDRPs are fully equipped to handle most complications and obstetrical procedures (sometimes even cesarean surgery). Both local and regional anesthesia can be used. The rooms can usually accommodate the parents, guests the parents may invite, physician or midwife, pediatrician, anesthesiologist, scrub nurse, circulating nurse, obstetric resident, and additional students.

As if contemporary hospital terminology weren't confusing enough, many hospitals do not make a distinction between the terms *LDR* and *birthing room*. For example, St. Mary's Hospital in Grand Junction, Colorado, a hospital where I observed maternity care for a few days, has a beautiful maternity unit known as the

Family Birth Center. It consists of six rooms (called birthing rooms) where the mother labors, gives birth, and spends the first postpartum hour or so. The mother then has the option of transferring to a mother-baby unit or going home. All mothers use these rooms despite risk status.

Hospitals with LDRs and LDRPs are eliminating the use of the delivery room for anything but operative obstetrics. For example, at the Birthplace in St. Mary's Hospital in Minneapolis, delivery rooms are open only for surgical birth, vaginal breech delivery, and multiple births. There are eighteen LDRP rooms, where the mother can remain from the moment she arrives to the time she goes home.

Requirements for using LDRs and LDRPs vary from one hospital to the other. However, the most common conditions either preventing the mother from using the room or leading to her transfer out of the room are: cesarean section, use of general anesthesia, presentations other than vertex (head-down), multiple births, and physician or client preference.

ADVANTAGES OF SINGLE-ROOM MATERNITY CARE

LDRs and LDRPs offer many advantages over the multitransfer system:

- ◆ *Increased safety.* Emergencies requiring immediate medical attention are handled more quickly, since there is usually no need to transfer the mother or newborn to another room. The risk of infection and injury during the move from one room to another is eliminated.
- ◆ *A smoother, less traumatic labor.* The laboring woman avoids the emotional trauma of moving from room to room, which can disrupt labor's progress.
- ◆ *Continuity of care.* The mother usually has the same nurses for labor, delivery, and the early postpartum period. There are fewer unfamiliar faces and therefore fewer emotional adjustments to be made.
- ◆ *A more positive birth experience.* Most parents greatly prefer remaining in a single homelike room throughout the childbearing process. When LDRP suites opened in one major Florida hospital, private patient deliveries increased

126 percent. Other hospitals have seen a similar increase in business after changing to a single-room system.

♦ *Low cost.* Using a single room for labor, birth, and the postpartum period is less expensive than transferring clients from labor to delivery to recovery to postpartum rooms throughout the childbearing experience. The multi-transfer system requires more personnel, more linen changes, more room and equipment cleaning. All these things increase the cost of both supplies and staffing. The hospital and ultimately the consumer will save money as single-room options become more popular.

ALTERNATIVE BIRTH CENTERS (ABCS)

To make terminology even more confusing, in some hospitals an *alternative birth center* (ABC) is another term for a birthing room. In others an ABC, also called a family birth center or twenty-four-hour suite, is a group of rooms for the family's use during the childbearing process. The ABC, or whatever you want to call it, is a childbearing center within the hospital. For example, the Family Birthing Center of Providence Hospital in Southfield, Michigan, is a freestanding childbearing center. It consists of very attractive single rooms where the family remains throughout labor.

The ABC represents what I consider the best option for hospital birth. ABCs may include a living room, small kitchen, and private bath, besides a birthing room. The family uses this space from admission to discharge, which usually takes place within twenty-four hours after the baby is born. Medical equipment is out of sight but readily available.

Routine medical intervention, such as the use of IVs and electronic fetal monitoring, is less common in the ABC than in other hospital settings.

The Alternative Birthing Center of Hillcrest Medical Center in Tulsa, Oklahoma, has a separate entrance. Parents don't feel as if they are entering a hospital with all its associations of illness. Each birthing suite consists of a private living room, family room, bathroom, and bedroom, and there's a kitchen families can share if they wish to prepare their own food. Parents can either bring their own food or order hospital food.

Today ABCs like this are rare, limited to disappointingly few hospitals throughout the world. The good news is that they are growing in number in response to consumer demand.

The Nursing Staff

The care the nurses provide, their attitudes, and their philosophy of childbirth greatly affect your birth. In the hospital a nurse or nurses will probably be more actively involved in your labor than your health care provider will be, unless your health care provider is one who remains with mothers throughout labor (as do many midwives and a few physicians). A nurse will check your baby's heart rate, your blood pressure, temperature, and pulse. In many hospitals nurses also do the vaginal exam to assess cervical dilation.

Nursing care varies widely from hospital to hospital. In some institutions a nurse remains with the mother throughout labor, providing one-to-one care; in others a nurse comes and goes to assess vital signs and labor's progress. Many mothers prefer to have a nurse present throughout labor. Others would rather be alone with their birth partner most of the time. If you want to be alone, simply tell the nurse that you and your partner would like privacy.

In a few hospitals nurses provide labor support as well as madical care. For example, at Bon Secours' progressive maternity unit in Grosse Pointe, Michigan, all the nurses are skilled in helping the mother with breathing patterns, guided imagery, and other comfort measures, and in helping the father to be involved in whatever way he wishes. Kathy Holland, RN and certified childbirth educator, says, "We are wholly committed to helping the mother and her partner achieve the kind of birth they want."

The Bon Secours nurses are eager to learn everything they can to better help mothers through labor. "We have discovered," Kathy Holland points out, "that the mind-over-labor method is far more effective in helping the mother cope with labor than focusing primarily on the breathing patterns. So we've all made the effort to learn it."

While observing nurses work with laboring mothers in hospitals throughout the United States, I have seen a surprising variation in nurses' outlooks on maternity care. In a few hospitals the entire maternity nursing staff embraces the ideas characterizing the *mind-over-labor* philosophy—namely, that childbirth is a normal process and the parents' right to the kind of birth they want should be respected. In other institutions nurses approach birth as a medical process and are unwilling or unable to meet the client's individual needs.

"I've found that many labor and delivery nurses have a tremendous amount of fear about birth," says Quila Rider, CNM, of Orange County, California, who conducts training programs for registered nurses. "Many foreign-trained nurses have told me that the American system with its emphasis on technology and malpractice suits scares the bejeebies out of them."

When you visit the hospital, meet the nurses to get an idea of their view of birth and style of maternity care. If you *have* to give birth in a hospital whose nursing staff does not share your view of childbirth, you can still achieve your goals, but you may have to work a little harder. Here are some suggestions:

- Pay extra attention to labor support. Consider hiring a labor support person to act as a consumer advocate.

- Provide the nursing staff with a copy of your birth options plan, signed by your health care provider.

- Meet with the head nurse or unit manager. Be specific and state precisely what you want for your birth.

- Be polite but firm about your position if, during labor, a nurse insists on a particular procedure you wish to avoid. If necessary, you or your birth partner can repeat your position. Don't be intimidated if asked to sign a waiver or consent form. This is a normal rule in many institutions if you refuse a routine procedure.

Planning a Hospital Birth

The major steps in planning a rewarding hospital birth experience are choosing a health care provider who supports your birth plans and choosing the best hospital in your area for your personal needs.

Consider hiring a childbirth companion to help you achieve your personal plans and provide additional emotional and physical support in the unfamiliar environment. A childbirth companion can go a long way toward helping you create the optimal hospital birth.

Before she became a CNM, Quila Rider worked with another woman, providing a childbirth companion service to women giving birth in hospitals. "My partner and I would meet with the woman to get to know her and help her develop a birth plan," she says. "The birth plan would include a statement of what she wanted in the birth. We would help her negotiate over a period of weeks or months, if necessary, with the hospital nurses, particularly the nursing supervisor, physicians, and sometimes even the perinatologist she might be visiting. We could get in writing a final birth plan signed by all appropriate persons. This was tremendously effective in helping parents achieve their goals."

CHOOSING THE BEST HOSPITAL

"People often ask us why we traveled so far for our child's birth and whether it was worth the inconvenience," says one mother who carefully chose her maternity hospital. "Traveling twice the distance would have been worth it. When you're in labor, you are hurt and scared. It is no time to fight for your rights. The staff supported our decisions rather than made us feel as if we were inconveniencing anyone. We were encouraged in a natural and gentle birth the way we wanted it."

Some parents choose their health care provider first, then select the hospital. Others select a hospital, then look for a health care provider who practices there. In either case, it is worth spending the time and effort to select the best possible birth setting in your area.

Here are some suggestions to make sure the hospital you choose is the best for you:

- ◆ Visit the hospitals in your area and talk to the staff before making a final choice. Meet with the staff to find out if they are committed to parent-oriented maternity care. This is more important than the physical setting. You can have a much more positive birth in a conventional room with sensitive staff who individualize their care than you can in a birthing room with staff who view the mother as an ill patient and who follow rigid policies.

- ◆ Formulate a verbal or a written birth plan specifying your wishes regarding health care options from labor to discharge. Hospitals vary dramatically in their routines and protocol. For example, even in birthing rooms mothers and newborns are sometimes separated. However, you can request that the infant exam and other newborn procedures take place while you and your mate hold the newborn.

♦ When you visit the hospital, ask questions to assess the birth place. Address your questions to nurses, the head nurse, or the unit manager. See the section in this chapter titled Questions to Ask the Hospital Staff.

♦ Find out the criteria for using the birthing room, LDR, LDRP, or ABC. As we have seen, in some hospitals only mothers considered low-risk may use these options. In others too-strict screening requirements exclude even perfectly normal women, such as those who are planning a vaginal birth after a previous cesarean. A few hospitals even require special birthing room classes!

♦ Find out about the criteria for transfer out of the birthing room, etc. Some hospitals have a high rate of transferring mothers out of birthing rooms and alternative birth centers to conventional labor and delivery rooms for minor or suspected complications as well as for medical emergencies. Some hospitals do not allow mothers to have pain-relief medication or Pitocin-augmented or induced labors in these more peaceful settings. Therefore, if in the midst of labor the mother feels she needs pain relief, or if her health care provider opts to use Pitocin, she must transfer.

♦ Be a shrewd consumer. Don't be misled by expressions like *progressive* and *family-centered maternity care*. Sometimes *progressive* refers only to a progressive policy about raising hospital income! The only way to know whether a hospital supports your view of birth is to visit the hospital, interview the staff, and talk with parents who have given birth there. It is utter folly to select a hospital without taking these steps.

♦ Find out about admission procedures before labor. Where possible, fill out papers in advance. Labor is no time for *either* parent to have to answer many questions and fill out forms.

WHAT TO LOOK FOR

While educating maternity care professionals, I have had the opportunity to participate in hundreds of hospital births throughout the nation. I've observed small hospitals with fewer than two hundred births a year and huge teaching institutions with ten thousand births yearly, hospitals with rooms ranging from simple and plain to worthy of elegant hotel suites. I think you should look for *all* the following characteristics when making your choice:

◆ *A safe environment for birth.* This includes an anesthesiologist available around the clock in case of an emergency cesarean section. There should be facilities to set up for surgery within no more than thirty minutes. For the mother with medical problems, a safe hospital may mean an acute care center.

◆ *Attractive and comfortable rooms.* Attractively furnished rooms are obviously more appealing and relaxing than sterile cubicles or rooms painted in clinical green. However, a birth place need not be beautiful if it is comfortable for you. One of the best and safest family-centered hospitals I have visited has simple, unadorned birthing rooms. But the nonintrusive health care and the staff's wholehearted commitment to serving individual needs more than made up for the lack of beautiful decor.

◆ *A staff who encourages the mother, not policy, to dictate the elements of her health care from admission to discharge.* You are the center of the childbearing drama. As one nurse puts it, "This means giving the mother complete control to the degree she wants to take it. If she wants to give birth standing up on the way back from the bathroom, that's what we help her do. We are here to support her choice, providing it does not endanger her or her baby's health."

◆ *A staff who welcomes the father (or birth partner) to remain with the mother throughout labor, birth, and the postpartum period, no matter where or how the phases occur.* The father should be welcome to remain through all procedures, including preoperative preparation for cesarean birth, administration of anesthesia, cesarean surgery whether or not the mother is awake, and the entire postpartum period. Most hospitals welcome the father during vaginal birth, but there are still a few that deny the father's right to witness the birth of his child if the mother has a cesarean, particularly if general anesthesia is used. "There is no excuse for this behavior," says obstetrician Dr. Donald Creevy, assistant professor at Stanford University School of Medicine. "No health professional, whatever his or her motive, should ever separate family members before, during, or after birth, no matter how the birth takes place."

◆ *A staff who view the father as an integral part of the family, never a visitor.* Many hospitals are making this distinction: visitors are limited to certain hours but fathers can remain with their family twenty-four hours a day if they want.

◆ *Flexible policies to better serve the family's needs.* Hospital policies vary widely. Some hospitals rigidly follow policy; in others, staff will bend policies to meet individual needs. For example, Chris Petrone, head of prenatal education at Manchester Memorial Hospital, says, "Individual flexibility underscores the basic philosophy of maternity care here. We recognize that families have individual needs and preferences, and we try to adapt to them rather than expecting them to accommodate us. The mother can give birth in the position of her choice; the father can deliver the baby if he wants, or he can cut the cord; children can attend births, surrogate parents can attend—whatever the parents want."

◆ *Freedom for the mother to invite the guests of her choice (family, friends, her children, labor support persons) to share her labor and birth.* The common excuse that there is no room or that guests will interfere with others' privacy is sheer nonsense. Most hospitals that deny a mother the company she wishes still find room for medical and nursing students to observe labor and birth.

◆ *Freedom for the mother to walk around as she pleases during labor.* Unless you have an unusual medical complication, you should always be free to move about. For many women, walking and remaining upright during labor hasten labor's progress and reduce discomfort.

- *Freedom for the mother to shower, take baths, or use the Jacuzzi as she wishes,* whether or not her membranes have ruptured. More hospitals now have bathtubs or Jacuzzis for laboring women. During active labor warm water can relax the mother, reduce pain, and often hasten labor's progress. Yet some hospitals restrict mothers with ruptured membranes from taking tub baths, on the theory that the risk of infection increases once membranes have ruptured. However, if you are in active labor, there will not be enough time for an infection to develop.

- *No routine medical procedures for the essentially healthy laboring woman.* Such procedures as shaving the perineal area, administration of an enema, intravenous feeding, continuous or intermittent electronic fetal monitoring, artificial rupture of the fetal membranes, and performing an episiotomy should not occur unnecessarily. (Obstetrical interventions and routines are discussed in chapter 4.)

- *Encouragement of breastfeeding.* The mother who plans to breastfeed should receive support to breastfeed exclusively. The baby should never receive bottles of formula or water without the mother's request.

- *No separation of healthy infants and mothers at any time throughout the hospital stay.* Though many hospitals advertise rooming-in, they often place infants in the nursery at certain times, such as during visiting hours.

- *Privileges granted to certified nurse-midwives.* Any hospital with the consumer's needs at heart will willingly grant privileges to CNMs. It may not necessarily have midwives on staff, as there may simply be no midwives practicing in the area. The important thing is that the hospital has an open door to midwives.

FAMILY-CENTERED MATERNITY CARE

Family-centered maternity care, or FCMC, is a philosophy of care that focuses on the psychological and social needs of the mother, father, newborn, and other family members and the physical needs of the mother. A hospital that truly embraces FCMC individualizes the mother's maternity care to meet her personal needs; fathers are welcome to be involved throughout the labor and birth process, no matter if the baby is born vaginally or via cesarean section; labor and birth take place in a homelike setting; no restrictions are placed on children participating during labor and birth, visiting their mothers, and interacting with their newly born sibling; and a program of early discharge allows the mother to adapt to the first few days of new parenthood in her own home.

Although it is a valid and important idea, FCMC can be a misleading term. For example, some hospitals claiming to be family-centered prohibit children from visiting in the first hours after birth, as if they were not part of the family! And a few will not allow fathers to attend cesareans, particularly if general anesthesia is used. Hospital birth is a competitive business, so many institutions advertise FCMC to attract clients even when their policies are inimical to the true meaning of family-centered care.

"Be wary of such places," warns Dr. Celeste Phillips. "Hospitals that separate family for *any* reason are not good places for childbearing."

In their book *Family Centered Maternity Care*, Professor Susan McKay and Dr. Celeste Phillips point out that: "comprehensive FCMC is not well-decorated birthing rooms with flowered wallpaper...nor is it birthing chairs or birthing beds....Restrictive policies and protocols often dominate care. In such settings, parents are 'allowed' to hold their baby, and siblings are 'permitted' to touch their new brother or sister only with physicians' orders and only during certain times. Such restrictions make it very obvious to the family just who is in charge, i.e., the professional staff."

QUESTIONS TO ASK THE HOSPITAL STAFF

The answers to the following questions can help you decide if a hospital is the right place for you and your baby. You can direct these questions to staff nurses, the head nurse on the birthing unit, or an administrator.

+ Is nursing care provided one-to-one? If not, how many laboring women does each nurse care for?
+ Are any medical procedures (intravenous feeding, continuous electronic fetal monitoring, and so forth) routine? If

continuous electronic fetal monitoring is not routine, is monitoring routine at any time during labor?

◆ If any procedures are routine, what percentage of mothers ask to have them waived?

◆ How does the staff react when a mother or father waives a routine?

◆ Do laboring women have a private bathroom? Shower? Bath?

◆ Is the mother free to shower or bathe during labor? Can she use the bathtub or Jacuzzi whether or not her membranes rupture?

◆ Is the mother free to eat lightly and drink liquids as she wishes during labor?

◆ Is the mother free to walk around as she pleases throughout labor?

◆ Can women give birth in the position of their choice?

◆ Are stirrups commonly used for delivery?

◆ What percentage of mothers use the birthing room?

◆ Are there any restrictions on using the birthing room? If so, what are they?

◆ What percentage of women transfer out of the birthing room? What are the most common reasons for transfer? (Look for a transfer rate of less than 5 or 6 percent.)

◆ Are fathers (or other birth partners) welcome to remain with the mother throughout all procedures, including preoperative administration of anesthesia, cesarean surgery, and postoperative recovery?

◆ May the mother invite whomever she wishes, including her children, to share her labor and birth?

◆ Do certified nurse-midwives have privileges?

◆ What is the cesarean rate? Ideally it should be 10 percent or less, but you'll be lucky to find a hospital with a rate less than 20 percent.

◆ Do most mothers breastfeed? Do breastfed babies routinely receive bottles of water or formula?

◆ Are healthy infants and mothers separated for any reason? At night? During visiting hours?

◆ How many mothers choose to go home within two to six hours after giving birth?

◆ If the mother chooses to stay in the hospital postpartum, does her baby remain with her twenty-four hours, even when she has visitors?

◆ Are children welcome to see and hold the healthy newborn within the first hour after birth?

◆ Can fathers room with the mother and baby twenty-four hours a day?

IF YOU ARE A HIGH-RISK MOTHER

Your pregnancy or labor may be labeled high-risk if you have previous medical, current obstetric, or social or economic conditions that are potentially dangerous to the health or life of you or your baby. The mother with a potentially complicated labor requires more watchful medical care and, often, medical intervention. The increased likelihood of special needs limits her options. For example, the mother who would benefit from intravenous medication or continuous electronic fetal monitoring may have less mobility and may not be able to give birth in the position of her choice.

However, all mothers—despite risk status—will benefit from giving birth in an emotionally positive climate where their psychological and physical needs are met. A supportive setting is especially important for the high-risk mother. During labor, such a mother often experiences feelings of failure, guilt, and anxiety. Being in a comfortable place, surrounded by family and supportive loved ones, can help her and her mate experience a positive birth even in the presence of complications.

In a few hospitals you as a high-risk mother have these options. For example, in the University of Utah Medical Center in Salt Lake City, mothers with medical complications are welcome to use the birthing rooms. A special high-risk birthing room adjoins a nursery.

The mother and baby with medical problems can benefit by eliminating the last-minute rush to the delivery room. As Dr. Richard Stewart says, "We don't transfer clients from one room to another if complications arise or the mother requests medication. If complications develop, the family remains with the mother."

Siblings of a high-risk infant can also benefit from being present during labor or in the immediate postpartum period. They should feel welcome to visit the sick newborn in the intensive care unit. This will enhance siblings' acceptance of the infant and will have a positive effect on the entire family.

It is heinous that in many hospitals only women who are likely to have perfectly normal deliveries are "candidates" for such options. As Susan McKay and Celeste Phillips point out, "Segregation of families so that some are eligible for family-centered intrapartum (labor) care while others are not is discriminatory and masks the goal of a family-centered program—that is, to provide for the needs of all family members, regardless of the specifics of the birth experience."

Some hospitals prevent siblings from visiting the sick infant. This policy stems from the bizarre belief that the presence of family will increase the risk of infection but has no basis in fact. Hospitals already have far more pathogenic (infection-causing) microbes than anyone is likely to bring in from outside. Besides, family members are just as capable of scrubbing their hands as medical professionals. Pioneer pediatrician John Kennell conducted a study showing that family members were even more careful about hand washing![5]

IF YOU CAN'T FIND AN IDEAL HOSPITAL CLOSE BY

Unfortunately, in some areas there are no hospitals that support the options every parent deserves. If this is the case in your area, you may still be able to plan the birth you want.

Many hospitals are ripe for change. For example, I am often invited to conduct workshops in hospitals whose nursing staff at first appear rigid in their views. Yet the nurses are eager to learn new ways to support the mother through labor, get the father involved in the childbearing process, and see hospital policies change.

In one hospital where I was to lecture, birthing rooms had replaced the combination labor and delivery room. However, women continued to remain in bed during active labor. I had given an all-day workshop for the staff and was preparing to give a talk to an auditorium full of expectant parents when the nurse manager of the laboring and delivery unit took me aside and said, "Tell them it's okay to get out of bed!"

"But I thought it was hospital policy...," I started to say when she snatched my arm. "That's why I can't tell them!" she said. "The doctors don't want to change. The only ones who can change this place are the parents and speakers like you!"

You may be able to plan the birth you want simply by asking for it. The maternity staff in some hospitals may welcome your request. However, it's best not to depend on this: some hospitals will refuse to deviate from policy.

To maximize your chance of a positive birth experience in a less-than-ideal situation, consider the following steps:

- Choose a health care provider who is as supportive as possible of your goals.

- Draw up a written birth options plan. Discuss your plan with the staff and be prepared to make compromises.

- Consider hiring a childbirth companion to deal with the staff and see that your birth plans are followed.

- You may even want to consider temporarily relocating to be near a hospital that offers more flexible birth options. Some parents have traveled to friends' or relatives' homes in other cities.

Resistance to Change

Creating change within the hospital is a long-term process. It means changing the attitudes of health care providers and nurses. For example, when the Birthplace at St. Mary's Hospital in Minneapolis was opened, many nurses had to develop a new view of the childbearing family. "The change was slow and painful," recalls head nurse Colleen Gerlach. A full third of the staff, who were unable to accept the change, found employment elsewhere.

When Dr. Richard Stewart conceived of the Douglas Birthing Center in Douglasville, Georgia, he at first faced tremendous resistance to his ideas. The main thing physicians opposed was Dr. Stewart's plan for midwives to do deliveries without a physician present. "Normal, healthy women with uncomplicated pregnancies need midwives, not doctors," he insisted.

Physicians also resisted Dr. Stewart's practice of discharging mother and baby within six to eight hours after birth. Now most health practitioners realize that early discharge enables mothers to make a smoother transition to parenthood. Nevertheless discharge within twenty-four to forty-eight hours is still the rule in many hospitals and childbearing centers across the nation.

Like the opposition to midwives and the prejudice against home birth, resistance to changes in maternity care rests on odd beliefs and emotions rather than on reason. Several factors contribute to the resistance:

- ◆ Some physicians and nurses find it hard to accept parent-directed maternity care and the lack of established routine. They are uncomfortable with the father's active role during labor, family and friends coming and going, and the mother's being able to walk around as she pleases and to give birth in the position of her choice.

- ◆ Parent-controlled birth requires viewing childbirth in an entirely different way than most physicians and nurses have been taught. The practitioner must reeducate herself about childbirth and learn to view the mother as a healthy client rather than an ill patient. This takes time.

- ◆ Some staff find the flexible policies hard to accept and to put into action. They are only familiar with one-size-fits-all maternity care and have difficulty accepting the needs of individuals with a variety of birth plans.

- ◆ Nurses with training and experience in obstetric technology sometimes find it difficult to work in a less intervention-oriented environment. The head nurse of one busy unit told me, "We used to believe that electronic fetal monitoring was beneficial with all patients despite risk status. Then studies showed that EFM could be hazardous with low-risk women. Conscientious practitioners discontinued routine EFM. Then we believed it could help the high-risk and even was mandatory for the high-risk. Now the studies show that EFM may be hazardous with high-risk. But the staff continues using the machine!"

- ◆ Some physicians find the contemporary birth settings less convenient for them. They prefer standing at the delivery table rather than stooping over a low bed to catch a baby.

With experience most health professionals learn to adapt to the philosophy and setting of contemporary hospital birth options. After having participated in many births, they discover that the new way is not only safe, but a more positive experience for the entire family and, therefore, more satisfying for the practitioner.

Susan Driesel, the head of the women's health center at Hillcrest Medical Center in Tulsa, Oklahoma, has seen a dramatic change take place in the attitudes of her staff: "Many physicians and nurses felt that 'new' birth options were unsafe, risky, and that there would never be a demand for the new style. It just didn't fit in with their paradigm. It didn't have a place in what they considered acceptable practice. When Hillcrest opened the Alternative Birth Center, physicians and nurses who were skeptical had the opportunity to witness the mothers receiving support. This gradually dispelled their fears. They could see freedom of mobility, the presence of support persons of the mother's choice, laboring without intravenous feeding or monitoring all working in that environment. They learned to accept these things and incorporate them into the traditional environment."

HOW YOU CAN HELP

Out-of-home birth continues to improve. Perhaps the day is not far off when every maternity hospital will have birthing suites.

One nurse manager sums it up: "It takes courage to change, to let go of old habits, sometimes to completely rethink what you have been taught, and to see the mother as a client who has the right to dictate to us what she wants (even if we don't agree). Many nurses just aren't willing to make that change. For them, there are other hospitals. But for those who choose to remain here and ride the change out, there is no turning back. You cannot experience contemporary birth options and ever want it any other way."

Who makes those efforts? You the consumer. Every parent who interviews hospital staff, carefully plans the birth, and refuses to compromise with unfair policies is contributing to a lower cesarean rate, a lower infant death rate, and a safer, more rewarding experience for all.

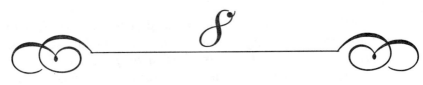

Birth in a Childbearing Center

Bridget's first child was born in a Los Angeles hospital. "There was nothing bad about the birth," she recalls. "It was just impersonal— a clinical experience. I felt as if I were on an assembly line. But I was like many women. I didn't know any better. Unless you've experienced something different, you may not even realize what you've missed. You may think hospital birth is the best there is."

The birth went well; mother and baby were healthy. However, Bridget knew there was something missing. When she was pregnant again, she discovered another way. Her next child was born in the Marchbanks Alternative Birth Center in La Habra, California.

"I never imagined how different labor could be," Bridget said. "The birthing center had a personal, loving, and caring atmosphere. I felt like I was the most special person on earth.

"There, having a baby wasn't just a woman's thing. The staff wanted my husband, my daughter, Tracy, and me to have the best experience. Dr. Marchbanks invited Tracy to be involved throughout. My family was also welcome. Besides my husband, my mother, sister, sister-in-law, my aunt, and my grandma shared the birth. The physician remained with me the whole time during labor and after the birth. It made me feel special.

"We plan to have another child. And the birth will be at the childbearing center. There's no comparing the two experiences."

A growing number of parents have made a similar discovery— especially those who have given birth in different settings. They frequently opt to give birth to their next baby in a childbearing center either because they were dissatisfied with their hospital

174

experience or attracted to the idea of giving birth in a more homelike setting with flexible policies.

What Are Childbearing Centers?

A childbearing center, also called a birthing, birth, or alternative birth center, is a homelike facility outside a hospital setting for prenatal care, labor, birth, and the first few hours after birth. Many centers are called *freestanding*, to indicate that they are physically, officially, and financially independent of a hospital. About 50 percent of birthing centers are nonprofit organizations. Corporations own some, and private physicians or midwives own others. Hospitals also own and manage many centers.

Birth centers are modeled on the home, not the hospital. Perhaps the major factor distinguishing childbearing center both from hospital birth is, in the words of one physician, "the feeling of giving birth at home away from home."

Though they vary from one center to another, birth center policies are far more flexible than those in most hospitals. As the National Association of Childbearing Centers (NACC) states, "Hospitals create policies to care for people who are sick, while freestanding birth centers design programs for healthy pregnant women."

In the birth center the laboring mother is able to wear her own clothing, eat and drink, shower or bathe, walk around as she wants, and invite her family, children, and the guests of her choice to share her birth. Most important, she, not the staff, is the center of the childbearing drama.

AN EVOLVING CONCEPT

Birth centers are relative newcomers to maternity care. They evolved in the 1970s primarily to meet the needs of many parents dissatisfied with traditional hospital delivery and home birth. According to Ruth Watson Lubic, general director of the Maternity Center Association, the hospital health care delivery system has failed for the most part to respond to the needs of childbearing families.

While home birth often meets the needs of the expectant

parents, the lack of skilled, experienced home birth practitioners in many areas left parents with either the traditional hospital, a home birth attended by a poorly trained midwife, or a do-it-yourself birth. Parents were actively seeking safe alternatives.

A few pioneer practitioners were willing to meet their clients' needs. For example, Howard Marchbanks, a pioneer physician who attends hospital, childbearing center, and home births, has been delivering babies in his own freestanding childbearing center in Southern California since 1973. Dr. Marchbanks is committed to helping clients create the birth of their choice. He believes the mother should have the option of choosing where her baby will be born.

Other pioneers include Victor and Salee Berman, who created the first California birth center and one of the first in the United States. Beginning with the desire to create a more humane experience for their clients within the hospital, they proposed a single room for labor, birth, and the postpartum period. Though such LDRP (labor, delivery, recovery, postpartum) rooms are now common throughout the nation, at the time the Bermans proposed their idea, it was considered too unconventional. They created a birth place within their OB-GYN office.

Though a few practitioners were providing a birth place for mothers in a homelike out-of-hospital environment, the Maternity Center Association (MCA) in New York City developed the first childbearing center accepted as a recognized part of the maternity health care system. The persons primarily responsible for this advance were certified nurse-midwives Ruth Watson Lubic, general director of the MCA, and the present director of the National Association of Childbearing Centers, Eunice Ernst. Ruth Lubic says parents "were engaging in do-it-yourself home birth rather than submit to in-hospital maternity care."[1]

MCA opened the Childbearing Center in Manhattan in September 1975 to provide safe maternity care sensitive to human needs at a lower cost than hospital care. MCA opted for opening the Childbearing Center instead of creating a home delivery system for several reasons. First, home delivery was more expensive for the practitioner. Second, home birth has potential dangers—not to the mother but to the practitioner traveling in New York City at odd hours of the night! As Ruth Lubic puts it, "Even in the mid-fifties, safety of staff traveling through the city at all hours had become a problem for Maternity Center Association's home birth service." MCA has since opened another birth center in New York, the Childbearing Center of Morris Heights in the South Bronx.

As with most major changes, birth centers were greeted with mixed reactions, ranging from enthusiastic applause to bitter condemnation. The latter stemmed primarily from physicians. Despite opposition, MCAs safe, out-of-hospital birth environment flourished. It has provided the inspiration that has changed the face of American childbirth forever.

Within a few months other freestanding childbearing centers opened throughout the United States. "We borrowed heavily from Ruth Lubic and the Maternity Center Association when we set up our birthing center here in Douglasville, Georgia," says obstetrician Dr. Richard Stewart. "They broke the ground for us." The Douglasville Birthing Center, opened in 1976, was the first in-hospital birth center in Georgia.

The childbearing center scene is in a constant state of flux. More childbearing centers are opening throughout the Untied States in response to expectant parents' needs. However, one-third or more of those that open soon close their doors. There are two reasons for this. Midwives or physicians without business skills open many birth centers. Some centers don't meet the clients' needs for which these unique facilities were originally designed, namely a homelike environment where the mother receives noninterventive midwifery care. They are more like minihospitals than birth centers.

Nevertheless, childbearing centers continue to open in response to the growing needs of expectant parents. Today hundreds of childbearing centers are scattered throughout the United States. And there is every reason to believe that they will continue to evolve and their numbers grow.

The Setting

A physician beautifully describes his vision of the ideal childbearing center this way: "An old house with three or four small separate living areas, each with its own kitchenette and bathroom with both shower and tub. Each living area should also have a separate musical facility so individual families can play the music of their choice during labor. The furnishings should include antiques or modern furniture made in the old style, an antique rocking chair for the mother to use during labor, and lots of braided rugs for that homey feeling. For the birthing bed, an eight-thousand-dollar piece of equipment such as those in some hospital birthing rooms is hardly necessary. A comfortable double or queen-sized bed with lots of pillows will suffice.

"Of course, the center should have a large yard with a play area for the children and a large playroom with toys to use in inclement weather. This way, children attending births won't feel sequestered in one area throughout labor.

"Full-time midwives should staff the birthing home. It matters little whether they are certified nurse midwives or direct-entry midwives as long as they are well trained and competent. To keep everything centrally located, all prenatal care should take place in offices out of sight and sound in a basement or first floor.

"There is no reason centers like this can't exist right on the hospital grounds and independent of hospitals."

Few of the childbearing centers are quite as lovely as this physician's description. Most do not have entire living areas for each family, but birthing rooms only. Most do not have a yard where children can play. However, many centers—whether in Victorian homes or modern single-story buildings—come close to this vision.

Most childbearing centers are renovated homes. An increasing number are in professional office space. One center is in an apartment high-rise. The majority are independent of hospitals. The best birth centers have two or more private, attractively decorated birth rooms. They usually have an ordinary double bed (rather than a narrow hospital-sized bed) or a special birthing bed designed to facilitate maternity care during labor and birth. Cots or convertible couches are usually available for the mother's guests.

Many childbearing centers also have kitchen facilities the parents and those attending the birth can use. Some families bring their own food and drinks and prepare their own meals. In the Family Birthing Center in Upland, California, owned by Dr. Michael Rosenthal, the new parents can order a gourmet meal delivered!

In addition, many birth centers have a family room, examining rooms, a Jacuzzi, spa, or oversized tub for the mother's use during labor, a classroom, a room with toys where siblings can play, and a lending library.

Approximately five thouand babies have been born since 1973 in the Marchbanks Alternative Birth Center in La Habra, California. Childbirth educator Barbara Mason, who radiates enthusiasm and inspires confidence in the parents' ability to give birth naturally, manages the two small but beautiful birthing rooms that the center offers. My wife, Jan, observed her first birth (other than her own) at the Marchbanks Center. The event was especially moving to me. For years Jan had been editing my published books but had never witnessed another mother's birth. She was with me on a lecture tour and we were staying at a hotel near the center when the phone rang at 7:00 A.M. A mother was in labor and we were invited to attend. I'll never forget the awe on Jan's face when she observed the birth of a baby girl. The room where the birth took place had a double bed and beautiful blue walls painted with clouds through which shone the rays of the sun—an appropriate and dramatic motif for a birthing room.

The midwife, Lorri Walker, RN, knelt at the foot of the bed while catching the baby. As the baby's head was born, Lorri gently massaged the perineum so the mother would not tear. When the head was born, Lorri guided the mother's hands to take the baby under the arms and complete her own birth as the father held his wife closely. This wonderful birth took place in a room suffused with a sense of peace.

Each room at this center has a soft cotton rope hanging from the ceiling like a vine. Many mothers find it helpful to hang on the rope while pushing. "It's amazing how this can help the descent of a baby during a difficult second stage," says Dr. Marchbanks.

The Birth Center in Houston, Texas, owned and operated by certified nurse-midwife Pat Jones, also has a similar homelike setting. It is in a two-story Victorian home with two birthing rooms. Each room has a large closet where medical equipment is stored. The rooms are attractively decorated to look like home bedrooms.

The first floor includes an office for prenatal exams, a large living room, and an eat-in kitchen clients may use at their convenience.

Family Born, an alternative birth center located about an hour and fifteen minutes drive from St. Louis in Perryville, Missouri, and owned and operated by certified nurse-midwife Elizabeth Clifton, is a remodeled home. Besides an office, kitchen, and bathrooms, the center includes a family room, a birth room with a spa where the mother can labor and give birth if she wishes, a big old-fashioned bed, and a wardrobe with medical equipment. Elizabeth Clifton points out that at Family Born most women don't use the bed to give birth. The majority feel more comfortable giving birth squatting on the floor over a sterile pad.

Jackson Memorial Hospital in Miami, Florida, sponsors a unique freestanding childbearing center. Jackson Memorial is a tertiary facility (a hospital that provides care for high-risk clients who require the most sophisticated type of medical and technical intervention). The Birth Center of Jackson is a lower-cost alternative to traditional hospital care for low-risk childbearing families. The center is on the tenth floor of a high-rise building which also has offices, hotel rooms, and apartments. It consists of six large bedrooms, each with an adjoining private bath, two examination rooms, an education room, a waiting room, and offices. Staffing the Birth Center are certified nurse-midwives, a registered nurse, licensed practical nurses, and secretarial staff.

Some birth centers are more flexible than others and will accept a broader range of clients. All provide safe maternity care outside the hospital setting. All provide settings conducive to eliciting the laboring mind response (see chapter 2). Consequently, they offer a positive birth experience for mother, father, and baby.

Health Care

"It's not so much the physical place that matters," says Dr. Marchbanks. "It's the philosophy behind the care clients receive that counts. That's what makes the difference between childbearing center and hospital birth."

As Eunice Ernst, director of the National Association of Childbearing Centers, puts it, "A birthing center, first, is a place for the practice of midwifery," that is, noninterventive maternity care whether provided by a midwife or physician."

The care available at most childbearing centers is usually based on the view that birth is a normal, natural event. In the center the mother and her mate have the right to choose how she will give birth and to actively participate in the childbearing process.

According to Dr. Marchbanks, "Here we celebrate pregnancy and wellness. We want to get the message out that the mother's body functions without medical intervention in the overwhelming majority of cases."

Speaking about a unique childbearing center in Menlo Park, California, Pamela Eakins, Ph.D., of Stanford University, expresses a similar idea: "The Birth Place views childbirth as a physical, emotional, social, and spiritual rite of passage for mother and baby. Only secondarily is childbirth seen as a medical event."[2]

Dr. Michael Rosenthal of the Family Birth Center in Upland, California, explains, "We take the term 'nonintervention' in a very literal sense. It often means that women give birth without me using my hands."

The childbearing center philosophy emphasizes taking part in one's maternity care. For example, in some centers mothers learn to test their own urine and record their weight at appointments. Fathers view the cervix and learn how to do abdominal palpations (to feel the fetal outline) and time the duration of contractions.

The health care offered during pregnancy, labor, and the postpartum period varies from one birthing center to another. Most, however, offer the following throughout the childbearing period:

- ◆ *Prenatal care.* Most centers offer prenatal care as well as care during labor. A few centers, however, provide health care only for labor, delivery, and the first postpartum hours. In this case the mother receives her prenatal care elsewhere, usually with the physician or midwife who staffs the center.

- ◆ *Care during labor.* In the best childbearing centers the mother receives warm, personalized care. Nursing or midwifery care is usually on a one-to-one basis. A good birth center can initiate emergency procedures in life-threatening situations and will have a backup hospital nearby with a system for rapid transport. In some birthing centers pain medication such as Demerol is available should the mother request it. In other centers the mother transfers to a nearby hospital if the need for pain medication arises. Bear in mind that the need for medication significantly decreases in the relaxing environment of the childbearing center.

The American Public Health Association's "Guidelines for Licensing and Regulating Birth Centers" recommend that labor shouldn't be stimulated or augmented with chemical agents such as Pitocin in the birth center setting.[3] Pitocin is used, however, in a few birth centers. For example, oxytocic drugs, intravenous feeding, sedatives, and narcotics are all available at the Alternative Birth Center in Jacksonville, Florida. Other stimulants to labor that are used in some birth centers include herbal preparations and acupuncture.

Whatever the maternity care includes, the focus is on meeting not only the mother's physical but also her emotional needs, greatly increasing the chance of a safe, positive birth experience. Why? Because the mother's emotions directly influence labor. I believe the major reason childbearing center care leaves parents with a far more positive perception of the birth experience than do most hospitals is that the birth center is conducive to eliciting the laboring mind response. When the mother is fully able to yield to the changes the laboring mind response entails, her labor is more likely to progress efficiently.

- *Postpartum care.* Mother and baby usually remain in centers for twelve to twenty-four hours after birth. Some centers request that the mother return within a few days after discharge for a brief checkup. A few centers arrange for a nurse or midwife to visit the mother in her home a few days after birth.

- *Additional services.* Many birthing centers also offer childbirth classes, new parents' support groups, well-child care, and women's health care.

THE HEALTH CARE PROVIDERS

In childbearing centers a variety of health professionals provide maternity care: certified nurse-midwives, obstetricians, family physicians, a midwife-physician team, or direct-entry midwives. Most commonly, certified nurse-midwives provide the care.

Obstetricians own and operate many centers. For example, Dr. Michael Rosenthal owns the Family Birthing Center in Upland, California, which has a staff consisting of around-the-clock registered nurses, two certified nurse-midwives, and administrative personnel. Childbirth educators teach classes in the center and a lactation consultant is available to give breastfeeding information and help. In the Birth Place, a nonprofit organization in Menlo Park, California, an obstetrician, family physicians, and certified nurse-midwives attend women in labor. Maternity nurses and trained assistants are on call twenty-four hours a day.

A few centers also employ childbirth companions. For example, the Washington Birthing Center in Fremont, California, across the street from Washington Township Hospital, employs childbirth companions as full-time staff members twenty-four hours a day. Everyone works as a team to support the mother and her family. Gail Fiock, a childbirth companion at Washington Birthing Center, describes her job: "In addition to giving labor support, our duties include paperwork, care of the linen, taking vital signs, cleaning and restocking the birthing rooms, and cooking for mothers and their families as needed."

The advantage of an on-staff childbirth companion is additional labor support for the mother. This spells reduced complications and shorter labors. Ideally the mother chooses her own labor companion and meets with her before labor.

Direct-entry midwives practice in a few childbearing centers. Even in states where lay midwifery is not officially recognized, a few maverick physicians will allow a skilled lay midwife to give prenatal care and deliver babies. However, given the questionable legal standing of lay midwifery, this fact is not advertised.

The Safety of Childbearing Centers

"The National Birth Center Study," published in the *New England Journal of Medicine*, shows that freestanding birth centers provide a safe alternative to hospital birth for healthy women with normal pregnancies. Scientists analyzed the experiences of 11,814 laboring women at 84 freestanding birth centers. The 1991 study concluded that "the infant mortality rate was as low as that found in studies of hospitals with similar low-risk mothers. Meanwhile, there was a higher degree of personal satisfaction among women who gave birth in childbearing centers."

Several factors contribute to the safety of childbearing center births:

◆ Prenatal screening helps identify problems that could predispose the mother to complications during labor.

◆ Skilled physicians or midwives staff birth centers.

◆ Equipment to handle medical emergencies is readily available.

◆ The mother receives individual care throughout labor.

◆ Most centers have a cooperative relationship with a nearby hospital in case a last-minute transfer is necessary. A system for rapid transport to the nearby hospital is also available.

A study of randomly selected mothers who chose childbearing center and home birth revealed that the majority felt in-hospital birth was as risky or more risky than birth out of the hospital. The risks they mentioned included infection, mother-infant separation, induced labor, surgical birth, and pressure about accepting excessive interventions including drugs.

The mother who plans a childbearing center birth should have good prenatal care and observe healthy dietary habits throughout pregnancy. In her practice in southern California, Lynn Amin, CNM, observes that "clients who don't follow a good diet, are obese, and who are not physically active are the ones most likely to have complications and transfer to the hospital."

Though health care providers carefully screen expectant mothers to increase the chance of a normal, healthy birth, this doesn't rule out all possibilities of complications. Such unusual complications as placental abruption (the placenta detaches from the uterine wall) occasionally arise. Remember, though, that there are also risks inherent in hospital birth. Many proponents of out-of-hospital birth feel that, for the healthy mother, the risks of birth in the hospital are greater than those of birth in the childbearing center.

An Enigma

The major reason mothers select childbearing centers instead of home birth is concern for safety. The impulse to leave home to give birth is one of the most peculiar and costly phenomena of modern times. *Unless the center is closer to a hospital than the mother's home, home birth is probably just as safe as long as the health care provider effectively screens the mother for risk and an experienced physician or midwife with medical equipment attends the birth.* When you consider it, the childbearing center is a billion-dollar industry founded on the curious belief that a healthy woman *needs* to leave her home to have a baby. Lynn Amin, a certified nurse-midwife who attends births both at home and in her childbearing center in Riverside, California, admits, "My heart is with home birth." She nevertheless opened a beautiful birthing center with a homelike environment because many of her clients were uncomfortable giving birth in their own homes. "Home birth is not widely accepted in the United States," she points out. "Many women, especially first-time mothers, are afraid to give birth at home. In this culture mothers are accustomed to go somewhere to have their babies. The childbearing center is becoming the place to go." What's the difference between the childbearing center and home? Ms. Amin says, "If they come here, I clean up. If I go to their house, they clean up!" This is the *only* difference between a home and a childbearing center birth.

Who Gives Birth in Childbearing Centers?

Childbearing centers vary in their criteria for accepting clients. In 1979 the American Public Health Association (APHA) adopted a set of guidelines for licensing and regulating birth centers, emphasizing that only mothers with normal, uncomplicated pregnancies should be clients.

Complications preventing mothers from giving birth in childbearing centers are similar to those ruling out home birth. These include maternal illness such as diabetes, chronic hypertension, complications of labor such as breech position, and premature labor.

Health care providers have different criteria for deciding just what is a low risk. The purpose of risk screening is to ensure the safety of mother and baby. No one-size-fits-all screening method is valid. In many centers, however, policies for risk assessment have become rigid. Many focus more on the policy than on the person. Some health care providers will not accept a perfectly healthy client simply because they feel the client belongs in some previously defined high-risk category. For example, many centers will not accept clients over thirty-five or under nineteen years of age or women who are planning a VBAC (vaginal birth after a previous cesarean). Providing the mother is healthy and there are no complications in this pregnancy, these women have the same chance of a safe, positive birth as anyone else.

Strict policies for accepting clients or transferring clients to hospitals are not always the fault of the childbearing center. Often, as Eunice Ernst points out, compromise is necessary: "In some areas, if it weren't for adapting certain policies, the childbearing center would never open."

As Dr. Richard Stewart of the Douglas Birthing Center, complains, "The medical community can be like a watchdog in making sure that you transfer every little complication. For example, if the mother loses 475 cc of blood postpartum, she may not be in any trouble or need anything. However, she fits the criterion for postpartum hemorrhage, which is a loss of greater than 450 cc, and therefore has to transfer. To have the medical community looking over your shoulder with such criticism and to have to observe every criterion to the letter is a pain in the butt."

The VBAC mother and others with special needs may benefit from the positive emotional climate of the childbearing center. Therefore, unless there are real medical complications during her present pregnancy, the option of childbearing center birth should be open to her.

Dr. Michael Rosenthal names risk assessment "the most important thing in deciding whom you are going to accept as a client." However, his idea of low risk is much broader than that of most physicians and midwives who run birthing centers. His birth center clients range in age from sixteen to forty-three, and he readily accepts VBAC mothers—even those who have had multiple cesareans. Between 1985 and 1990, 154 VBAC mothers have given birth in his Family Birthing Center without complications.

Childbearing centers that are close to hospitals, however, can take clients at greater risk. The Family Birth Center is only 150 yards from a hospital. "This allows us to be more flexible about our clients than we might be if we were five miles from a hospital," Dr. Rosenthal points out. Many birthing centers will not accept clients in labor who are more than two weeks preterm. Dr. Rosenthal, on the other hand, will accept clients four and five weeks preterm. "If a baby needs time in an intensive care nursery," he says, "we simply walk the baby across the street to the hospital. Should an emergency requiring a cesarean section arise, a client transfers to the hospital and is in surgery in less time than many hospitals can set up for surgical birth."

Ironically, while childbearing centers close to hospitals can safely accept clients at greater risk of a complicated labor, birth centers owned and operated by hospitals often have the strictest screening criteria of all. I believe that as the years pass, however, and practitioners gain more experience in these birthing environments, we will see increasingly relaxed criteria for accepting clients.

The Maternity Center in El Paso, Texas, a nonprofit organization founded by independent midwife Shari Daniels, was unique. (Unfortunately, it has closed its doors.) It consisted of a renovated old home in downtown El Paso where even high-risk mothers unacceptable to other birth centers could give birth. Very few risk factors in a woman's medical and previous pregnancy history spelled automatic refusal. Women from ages thirteen to fifty-one, those with a history of multiple cesareans, mothers with breech presentations, and mothers of twins all gave birth successfully in this center. The only grounds for automatic refusal of care at the initial application was an unwillingness to breastfeed.[4]

Childbearing centers vary in their criteria for accepting clients. Some birth centers will not accept a woman who has one or more of the following conditions.

Conditions Relating to Past Pregnancies and Births

◆ Grand multiparity (usually seven or more previous births; in some birth centers the mother with three previous births is classed as a grand multiparity)

- Previous cesarean section
- Previous premature birth (usually two or more previous premature births)
- Rh sensitization
- Incompetent cervix (that is, the cervix dilates before labor's onset)
- Previous birth to an infant with severe congenital abnormality, such as cerebral palsy
- Previous difficult vaginal delivery
- Previous stillbirth
- History of three or more miscarriages
- History of postpartum hemorrhage

Current Medical Conditions

- Chronic hypertension
- Such maternal illness as diabetes mellitus, epilepsy, renal disease, thyroid disease, heart disease, pulmonary disease, and sickle-cell disease
- Severe obesity
- Drug addiction and alcohol abuse

Conditions of the Current Pregnancy

- Excessive or inadequate weight gain
- Preeclampsia
- Significant vaginal bleeding
- Anemia
- Multiple pregnancy
- Premature labor (occurring before thirty-seven weeks' gestation)
- Postmature labor (occurring after forty-two weeks' gestation)
- Malpresentation (baby in other than the vertex or head-down position)

- Prolonged rupture of membranes (greater than twenty-four hours without labor's onset)
- Intrauterine growth retardation
- Polyhydramnios or oligohydramnios (too much or too little amniotic fluid)
- Active herpes infection at the time of labor
- Syphilis
- Such infectious disease as toxoplasmosis or rubella
- Placenta previa (placenta obstructing the cervical opening)
- Placental abruption
- Such other diseases of pregnancy as hyperemesis gravidarum (severe persistent vomiting)
- Any other condition for which hospitalization may be advisable

The Pros and Cons of Childbearing Center Birth

"After my first birth in the hospital I felt drained and exhausted," says an Oregon mother quoted by the National Association of Childbearing Centers. "I couldn't get any rest there for three days. At the birth center I delivered at ten A.M. and was sitting on my front porch rocking my baby at five P.M. I felt exhilarated and terrific. What a difference the care makes!"

The childbearing center provides an ideal setting for an increasing number of parents throughout the world for several reasons:

- The childbearing center is specifically associated only with pregnancy and birth. Unlike hospitals, childbearing centers are not illness-oriented, and they therefore provide a welcome alternative to the hospital setting.
- The health care provided at most birth centers is noninterventive. Though expert medical care is available and at most birth centers medical equipment is nearby, the emphasis is on the normality of labor.

◆ The childbearing center provides a setting for parents who are not comfortable with home birth yet don't want to give birth in a hospital. Many mothers *feel* safer in the birthing center. Feeling more secure enables many women to better surrender to labor and therefore to labor more efficiently.

◆ Childbearing centers offer personalized maternity care. Practitioners in most birth centers will individualize the care they provide to meet the parents' desires as long as nothing compromises the health of mother or baby. "We invite parents to ask questions and express their preferences," says Dr. Marchbanks. "There are almost no rules here that can't be broken to meet a mother's or family's needs."

◆ In most childbearing centers the clients can meet the entire staff before the birth. "We all become friends," says Lynn Amin of the clients at her center in Riverside, California. The expectant parents meet her backup and any of the nurses who may be attending. In larger centers, that staff nurses around the clock, clients are rarely able to meet the entire staff.

◆ The mother has a reduced chance of a cesarean section. The National Birth Center Study showed that the cesarean rate of nearly twelve thousand mothers who gave birth in childbearing centers was 4.4 percent, whereas the United States' cesarean rate as a whole is 27 percent. Of course, the national rate includes mothers at high risk while most birth centers include only low-risk clients. Nevertheless, even low-risk mothers are at increased risk of cesarean surgery in traditional hospitals because of common medical interventions. For example, one study compared a matched group of 250 low-risk mothers delivering in Jackson Memorial Hospital in Miami, Florida, with a matched group of mothers giving birth at the Birth Center of Jackson, located across the street. The cesarean rate among the birth center mothers was 6 percent, less than half the hospital's rate of 14 percent.[5]

◆ Childbearing centers offer maternity care at a significantly lower cost than the traditional hospital, though far greater than the home. Cost of prenatal care and birth in childbearing centers varies, depending on the area. Most major medical insurance policies, including Medicaid and Champus (Civilian Health and Medical Program of the Uniformed Services) cover prenatal care and birth in childbearing centers. Since not all insurance companies cover home birth, this makes the birth center more attractive to many parents.

◆ Like home birth, childbearing center birth offers greater control of the birth experience, the mother's freedom to do whatever she wants during labor, the parents' freedom to invite whomever they want to their birth, and the comfort of laboring in a nonclinical setting.

Bear in mind that not all of these benefits are available in every birth center. Some centers have rigid policies and less-than-ideal maternity care. However, the benefits described above are available at most birth centers.

The few disadvantages of childbearing centers vary from place to place:

◆ Although childbearing centers have more flexible policies than hospitals, the mother is still not on her own turf as she would be at home. She is, in essence, paying for a home birth away from home.

◆ Childbearing centers are not available everywhere.

◆ Rigid screening criteria often eliminate the perfectly healthy mother.

◆ Many childbearing centers have rigid rules requiring mothers to transfer to hospitals for conditions that could just as well be handled in the childbearing center.

Another potential disadvantage is that as childbearing centers become increasingly popular and physicians opt for giving care in centers to keep up with the competition, the childbearing center may become more like a hospital than a home. This has already happened at many centers where rigid policies and protocol rule. Dr. Michael Rosenthal points out, "Childbearing centers owned by obstetricians frequently fail because the doctors insist on practicing obstetrics rather than midwifery."

Benefits of a Childbearing Center Birth

Absence of restrictive policies
- Noninterventive maternity care
- The mother's freedom to invite the guests of her choice
- Reduced risk of a cesarean section
- Reduced need for pain-relief medication
- The freedom to give birth in the position of choice
- The freedom to eat and drink during the labor
- A homelike environment associated with childbirth, not with illness
- Reduced cost in comparison with hospital birth
- A more positive birth experience

Choosing a Childbearing Center

In most areas your choice of childbearing center is limited to the center closest to your home. In some cities, however, you may have several choices. For example, there are more childbearing centers in the Los Angeles area than in all of New England!

To find a childbearing center, check the yellow pages. Ask a childbirth educator if there are any centers within a reasonable drive of your home. You can also contact the National Association of Childbearing Centers (NACC) at (215) 234-8068 or write to RFD 1, Perkiomenville, Pennsylvania 18074 and ask for a list of childbearing centers. Enclose a self-addressed stamped envelope.

Here are some suggestions to help you make sure the birth center you choose is right for you:

- Visit the center. Meet and talk with the staff. The ideal childbearing center should be a homelike environment where you feel that you—not the staff—are the center of the childbearing drama.

♦ Learn about its policies. Do they agree with your birth plans? Most centers have flexible policies. Within reason, you can do just about anything you want. However, as previously noted, restrictive policies and a clinical-appearing environment make a few childbearing centers more like minihospitals than home.

♦ Find out about transfer criteria. For what reasons are most mothers transferred to hospitals? Some centers are more stringent in transfer policy than others.

♦ Find out how close the birth center is to a hospital, in case transfer is necessary. Visit the hospital to become familiar with its environment and polices.

♦ Find out what maternity care is available at the center. Are you given prenatal care at the center? Postpartum care?

When you have selected a childbearing center, discuss your birth options plan with your health care provider.

Transfer to a Hospital

A mother may transfer from childbearing center to hospital for a variety of reasons. These include slow progress during labor, prolonged first- or second-stage labor, fetal distress, maternal hemorrhage, and other complications. A baby may transfer if medical complications such as breathing difficulty make immediate pediatric attention necessary.

One woman in six of the 11,814 in the National Birth Center study transferred to the hospital. This, in my opinion, is a very high rate of transfer, and it is far higher than the transfer rates in some individual centers.

By comparison, only one in twenty at the Marchbanks Alternative Birth Center transfer. The major reason is maternal exhaustion after a prolonged labor. Similarly, at the Baltimore Birth Center (staffed by certified nurse-midwives) about 7 percent transfer, most often for lack of progress in labor. Often the mother suggests going to the hospital after a long labor. "Transfer is always a joint decision between the mother and her midwife," says Ann Sober, the registered nurse who manages the center. Generally speaking, the rate of transfer in hospital-owned centers is higher than that in freestanding childbearing centers.

Medical complications requiring hospital attention sometimes make transfer necessary. For example, one mother at the Family Birth Center in Upland, California, had a prolapsed cord (a grave complication in which the umbilical cord precedes the baby in the birth canal, cutting off the baby's oxygen). She transferred to a hospital across the street for an emergency cesarean section; the baby was born healthy.

Some centers require transfer to the hospital if the mother requests pain-relief medication or requires such medical intervention as intravenous feeding for dehydration or Pitocin to augment contractions. Others provide pain-relief medication and intravenous therapy as needed right in the center.

In my opinion, many mothers transfer unnecessarily. For example, a major reason for transfer is prolonged labor. However, if the mother isn't exhausted and the fetal heart tones are normal, she can try a variety of methods to get labor going again, including guided imagery, walking around, showering, bathing, nipple stimulation, lovemaking, or simply resting. If none of these methods works, then she should consider a transfer.

Several studies have shown so-called arrested labor to be another major reason for transfer. In this condition the cervix stops dilating for two or more hours or simply dilates slowly. Sometimes this is a genuine complication resulting from fetal malposition, cephalopelvic disproportion (the head is thought to be too large for the maternal pelvis), prior cervical surgery, or other factors. In other cases, however, the cervix simply dilates slowly. This doesn't mean labor is abnormal. Labor may stop for several hours and still be perfectly normal. Providing the mother and the baby are healthy, this is not a good reason for transfer.

In some birth centers mothers even transfer for prolonged early labor (that is, before the cervix is four or five cm dilated). Yet it is perfectly normal for a mother to be in latent labor with on-and-off contractions for two days or more. Rather than transferring to the hospital, she can simply go home until her labor becomes more active.

Still another inadequate reason for transfer is that the mother's membranes have been ruptured for more than twelve to twenty-four hours (the time depends on the center) without progress in her labor. The mother with ruptured membranes who is not in labor is often taken to the hospital for labor induction or augmentation to avoid the risk of infection. For example, Emily, a New Jersey mother of two, wanted to give birth to her first child in a birth center. However, her membranes ruptured and the baby was not born within twenty-four hours, so she transferred to a hospital. The experience was so disappointing that she decided to give birth to her second child at home.

Instead of transferring, the mother can remain where she is while her health care provider monitors for signs of infection. "If the mother's membranes rupture and she isn't having contractions," says Dr. Marchbanks, "we ask her to take her temperature every two or three hours. We don't do any vaginal exams, which can greatly increase the chance of infection. If the mother has no signs of infection, there is no reason she should transfer to the hospital."

There is little doubt that the transfer rates at many childbearing centers are much too high. However, mothers who transfer—for whatever reason—are often still glad they chose the childbearing center. Many express appreciation for the care in the center up to the time of and during the transfer.

Looking Ahead

The primary feature that makes childbearing centers special—and more attractive than hospitals to an increasing population—is that the childbearing center is more like a home than a medical facility.

In the future I hope we will see more childbearing centers for both high- and low-risk mothers. High-risk mothers are just as much in need of the emotionally positive climate the childbearing center offers as everyone else. Given their greater chance of developing complications, they are even more in need of a peaceful, homelike setting.

In the birth center the emotional tension of the hospital—where health professionals often anticipate problems—is absent. The setting is not only relaxing, it is positive and parent-centered. The care varies with the mother's wishes, not medical protocol. As Dr. Rosenthal puts it, "There is more touch than technology."

Conditions Requiring Mother's Transfer to a Hospital

Childbearing centers vary in their transfer criteria. Many will transfer mothers only for the more severe of the following conditions:

- Development of hypertension
- Malpresentation (baby in other than vertex or head-down position)
- Prolonged rupture of membranes
- Premature labor
- Any problem requiring forceps delivery or cesarean
- A request by mother for pain-relief medication or anesthesia, or the mother's need of intravenous feeding or Pitocin to augment labor
- Meconium staining of the amniotic fluid
- Abnormal fetal heart rate or pattern
- Lack of progress in labor
- Prolonged labor
- Cephalopelvic disproportion (the baby's head appears too large for maternal pelvis)
- Prolapsed cord
- Placental abruption (the placenta detaches from the uterine wall during pregnancy or labor)
- Placenta previa (the placenta partially or fully overlies the cervix)
- Maternal fever greater than 100.4° F
- Extensive lacerations
- Retained placenta
- Maternal bleeding
- Any other condition requiring medical treatment or observation

Conditions Requiring Newborn's Transfer
to a Hospital

After birth the baby may be transferred from the childbearing center to the hospital for any of the following reasons:

◆ Apgar score of less than 7 at five minutes after birth
◆ Abnormal vital signs
◆ Signs of pre- or postmaturity
◆ A congenital abnormality
◆ Respiratory distress
◆ Low birth weight, jaundice, or any other condition requiring medical treatment or observation

The sense of frustration, of not participating in one of life's most precious experiences, and the feelings of failure so common among mothers who give birth in traditional hospitals are rare among birth center mothers. Women leave centers with a feeling of satisfaction. The overwhelming majority of mothers (98.8 percent) included in the National Birth Center Study said they would recommend birth centers to their friends. Ninety-four percent said they would use the center during future pregnancies. Even among the mothers who transferred to hospitals, 96.9 percent said they would recommend childbearing centers to friends.

In childbearing centers women are *giving birth*; they are not having their babies *delivered*. It is for this reason, I believe, that the future of childbirth in the United States and in many other nations throughout the world lies with home birth and childbearing centers.

Birth at Home

Our first son, Carl, was born in a hospital where my wife, Jan, had first-rate medical care. The obstetrician who attended the birth, Leo Sorger, is a prominent and highly skilled New England physician. He is also one of those rare physicians who is fully committed to helping parents give birth the way they choose. The dimly lit room where Carl was born was peaceful, pleasant, and comfortable. The birth was a peak experience of our lives.

Nevertheless, we selected a home birth for our next child. Despite our positive hospital experience, we couldn't dismiss the fact that leaving our comfortable home in the middle of the night to go to a place associated with sickness had been unnecessarily traumatic. Beginning a family is a tremendously emotional time for the new parents—to say nothing of the baby. We felt we should experience it at home.

When our second son was born, we were living in an apartment in Brookline, Massachusetts. Since our apartment never quite felt like home, we rented a house on a hill in central Vermont for his birth. There, I caught our son Paul, as Dr. Thurmond Knight, a now-retired family physician, played Renaissance flute while waiting to help if necessary.

Jan was far more at peace in our rented home than she had been in the hospital. "I felt more comfortable and more secure. Also, it was wonderful to be able to stay in one place throughout labor."

Just a few miles from our rented home was a hospital that had the most consumer-oriented birthing units I had yet visited. However, we still chose to give birth in our mountaintop retreat. Later I discussed our decision with Dr. Louis DiNicola, a Vermont pediatrician who cares about mothers having joyful birth experiences and healthy babies. When I told him I thought our rented home was more comfortable than the hospital, he exploded: "You can't tell me that your rented house high on the top of that hill— where you are surrounded by snow and ice, where it's twenty below zero and the wind howls, where you have no central heating and you have to get up during labor to stoke up the stove with more wood—you can't tell me *that* is more comfortable than our birthing rooms! I won't accept it! Here you have all the conveniences of home. You don't have to be concerned about changing the sheets and cleaning up. We provide everything you need, including absolute privacy. And you don't have to worry about medical help if you need it. I simply can't believe that the place you and your wife chose to give birth is more comfortable in any way!"

He had a point.

I ended up rushing to the hospital shortly after Paul was born anyway. His brother, Carl, aged two years, two months, woke up shortly after the birth. In his excitement to greet his new brother, he dove across the room like an uncoiling spring and hit his head on the bed rail. The swelling was so immense that I thought it best to have it checked out.

If Jan had given birth in the birthing room, she could have had the same noninterventive care, the same peace and quiet. I could have caught the baby. The physician could have played the flute. Carl could have bumped his head on the hospital bed. And we could even have had a view of ancient sugar maples outside the window.

Yet there was a difference. Our rented home was *our* place—at least for the duration of our stay. It had a personal ambience—a sense of peace, comfort, and security—that no hospital could reproduce. Not even with a view of sugar maples.

When it was time for the birth of our third son, Jonathan, we decided that, since our Brookline apartment was our real home (like it or not), we would have the baby there. We hired Sloane Crawford, CNM, a Brookline midwife who helps parents plan the birth of their choice.

Few hospitals are as noisy as our bedroom was that Sunday morning between 4:00 and 5:00 A.M. Our apartment was on the second floor. During Jan's labor our downstairs neighbor (upset about being woken) began shrieking, hollering, swearing, and pounding on the walls. He finally called the police to complain about the noise! (It may have been in retaliation for my phoning the police many times about his loud stereo.) So besides the noise, we had unexpected company. I remember the face of a policeman who came to our apartment. He arrived just after the baby was born, and though he missed the birth, his face all but radiated with that near-magical glow I often see on the faces of people who witness their first birth. As he was leaving, he said to his partner, "A baby! It was just born!"

Despite the noise, interruptions, and visitors, comparing the two home births with our hospital experience, Jan recalls, "It was more peaceful, more relaxing, better to have the family together, and better in every way to be at home."

Thousands of parents agree. Parents who have had both hospital and home births invariably describe birth at home as a more positive experience. As one mother puts it, "There is simply no comparison. Hospital and home birth don't even belong in the same category!"

Birth at home was so important to Donna, a first-time expectant mother, that she traveled out of state because she couldn't find a physician or midwife to attend her home birth near the Florida town she lived in. She temporarily relocated to her grandmother's house in Alabama, where a midwife attended her birth. She describes her experience: "I was able to give birth in the same bed where my grandmother gave birth to all her five children, including my mother. Everyone in the room was crying tears of joy, but the tears that touched me most were my husband's as he held me and his baby boy. Mark and I lay in the clean bed with our brand new baby boy curled up between us, his little toes tucked under his little nightgown that I had made for him. We just couldn't go to sleep. We lay there for thirty minutes talking about the birth and about how happy we were. We couldn't wipe the smiles off our faces. It was so sweet and gentle and special. I wish I had a picture of that scene, although the picture will never leave my mind."

The Safety of Home Birth

Before the turn of the century, 95 percent of Americans gave birth at home. By 1940 only half the population was still giving birth outside hospital settings. By 1990 only 2 to 3 percent of U.S. mothers gave birth in their own home. Today home birth is again becoming the birth place of choice for an increasing number of parents.

Ann and Dennis, who chose home birth for both their children, echo the conclusion of other home birth parents: "After much research we felt we would be safer at home."

As Phillip G. Stubblefield, M.D., associate professor of Obstetrics and Gynecology of Harvard Medical School observes, "If the mother can be transported to a hospital within ten minutes where a team awaits capable of performing an emergency cesarean section, the outcome of an emergency at home may be better than if the mother were laboring in a small hospital where it would take half an hour to assemble the cesarean section team. In addition, there is evidence that at the extreme, the cold, overly professional atmosphere of the worst hospital settings may increase obstetric casualties."

Though research on the safety of home birth is limited, the few published studies have shown that for selected, healthy mothers, home birth is associated with lower cesarean rates, fewer complications, and optimum family-infant bonding.

In 1976 Dr. Lewis Mehl and his associates compared 1,046 home births with the same number of hospital births. The researchers matched both groups for maternal age, length of pregnancy, number of past births, risk factors, education, and socioeconomic status. There was no difference in infant mortality between the two groups. However, among the hospital births, there were significantly more cases of intrauterine fetal distress, elevated blood pressure during labor, lacerations, postpartum hemorrhage, birth injuries, neonatal infection, and babies in need of resuscitation. In the hospital, mothers used pain-relief medication more readily. There were more forceps deliveries and *nine times* as many episiotomies. These complications may have been iatrogenic, that is, physician-caused. They may have resulted from obstetric intervention and perhaps the hospital environment.[1]

In another study Dr. Mehl and his associates compared planned home births attended by midwives with physician-attended, planned hospital births. He matched the mothers for age, education, number of pregnancies, length of gestation, presentation (baby's position in relation to the mother's pelvis), and risk status. The researchers found no significant differences in perinatal mortality, birth weight, or other major complications. However, the home births were associated with higher Apgar scores (a test of the baby's color, pulse, respiration, muscle tone, and reflexes), less fetal distress, fewer incidents of postpartum hemorrhage, fewer birth injuries, and less need for infant resuscitation.[2]

Working with psychotherapists Gayle Peterson and P. H. Leiderman, Dr. Mehl also found that unmedicated home birth may have an improved psychological maternal outcome over anesthetized hospital birth: "Anesthetized hospital delivery was found to have a humiliating effect with decreases in self-worth and self-esteem, whereas natural hospital birth and more so, home delivery, tended to increase self-worth and self-esteem. More symptoms of postpartum depression were present in anesthetized hospital deliveries and decreased in the continuum from an anesthetized hospital to home delivery."

An extensive analysis of over thirty-two hundred births attended by Arizona's licensed midwives over the past eight years also shows impressive results. The perinatal mortality rate was 2.2 per thousand, including three deaths resulting from congenital abnormalities. Researchers Deborah A. Sullivan and Rose Weitz, associate professors of sociology at Arizona State University, state that this analysis, though not conclusive, "does suggest that there is little, if any risk involved in choosing midwife-attended out-of-hospital birth in Arizona."[3]

In the Netherlands—a country with one of the world's lowest infant mortality rates—about half of all births take place in the home. Home birth is more common in the Netherlands than in the United States because the Dutch accept it as normal. Midwives carefully screen mothers for risk factors, and emergency backup is always ready should it be needed.

Despite the evidence, many parents and professionals still believe that hospital birth means increased safety for mother and child. Historically, there *was* a dramatic reduction in maternal and fetal mortality when the place of birth shifted from home to hospital in this country. However, this does not mean that the hospital itself was responsible for the improvement. Other factors—better prenatal care, better nutrition, fewer low-birth-weight babies, the availability of antibiotics, and better diagnosis of complications—played a role in the improved outcome.

Misleading information about home birth continues to sway both professionals and the public. For example, in 1978 the American College of Obstetricians and Gynecologists (ACOG) issued a news release that claimed, based on information from eleven state health departments, that the risk to the baby's life was two to five times greater in out-of-hospital birth than in hospital birth.[4] Another study published in the *American Journal of Obstetrics and Gynecology* has given similar statistics. However, *neither of these studies distinguished between planned and unplanned out-of-hospital births.* Unplanned out-of-hospital births include late miscarriages, premature births, precipitous (that is, sudden, unplanned) deliveries, and unattended home births. Most of the unplanned births were precipitous deliveries. This complication is associated with about a seven-times-greater incidence of low birth weight, which in turn is associated with increased perinatal mortality. A world of difference separates a planned home birth from an emergency delivery in the car!

Does home birth present any risk? Unexpected life-threatening complications *do* occur during home birth. There is always an element of risk. Home birth carries a risk for both mother and baby. Acute emergencies like maternal hemorrhaging or fetal asphyxia can arise during labor and delivery without warning, requiring immediate medical attention that is not always possible at home.

For healthy mothers the risk is small. However, as home birth practitioners Drs. Stanley Sagov and Clara Feinbloom point out, "Families must be informed of this very small but real risk, which they must balance against the risks, largely iatrogenic and psychological, incurred in the hospital."[5]

No one can tell a mother she is perfectly safe giving birth at home. Whether she is safer at home than in a hospital, however, is another question. I'll always remember what one obstetrician (who practices in both hospital and homes) told me when Jan and I were considering whether to give birth at home. "If you ask me if home birth is a risk, I have to say yes. If you ask what I would do if it were my own child's birth, my answer would be 'Give birth at home.'"

Which is what we did.

The Pros and Cons of Home Birth

Anne's first child was born in a military hospital. After giving birth, Anne and her newborn were apart for twelve hours. For the next three days she saw her baby only once every four hours for bottle feedings. It was a frightening and painful experience for her.

Her second child was born twelve years later in a mountain home in Oregon. When she was pregnant with her third child, she planned for the birth to take place at home, but because of complications, she had to transfer to a hospital. The staff was overbearing. Again she felt totally powerless in a hospital environment.

"I wanted to create the most positive and supportive birth possible for my fourth child," she recalls. She had read about experienced waterbirth midwives in Hawaii. Excited about the possibility of having a waterbirth herself, she and her family packed their bags and moved to Maui. "We were blessed, finding a house and a midwife quickly. I began my nest arranging six weeks before my due date."

Once in active labor, she slipped into the tub. Near the time of birth, her husband and two of her other children also got into the tub. The baby was born into the warm water. Anne remembers, "My two-year-old stood next to me on the low seat and was the first to speak: 'That's my baby.'"

Anne gently lifted her baby to the surface, bringing her to her breast. "A few sputters, a muffled whimper, and she was breathing. I slid her back into the warm water. She was content to lie back, accustomed to the weightlessness and warmth of the water. I cradled the back of her little head in my palm. She floated, arms outstretched, eyes wide, calmly taking in her new home. We sat together, a bond of warm water flowing around and between us."

Anne's six-year-old son had stayed with her throughout the labor. After the birth he patted her on the back and said, "That was a great birth, Mom!"

Parents elect to give birth at home for many reasons.

For Kathy Kangas, who later founded Childbirth Education Services in Worcester County, Massachusetts, it was dissatisfaction with the hospital where she had given birth to her first child, Amanda. "Even though we carefully chose our obstetrician and discussed what I wanted—no IV, no monitor, no episiotomy, and so on—when we got to the hospital, it was a major war to get what I wanted. So when my husband, Tyler, and I got pregnant the next time, our first inclination was to give birth at home. I began to study about childbirth. It wasn't long before I knew staying home was not only more comfortable but safer, and that it was a risk to go to the hospital and get all that intervention or have to fight not to have it."

"Home birth," says Dr. DiNicola, "is a symptom of the failure of the medical profession to provide appropriate care for healthy mothers and babies. In hospitals almost everything is done for the convenience of the physician and delivery room personnel, not for the comfort of mother and child." While dissatisfaction with hospital birth is a primary reason parents choose to give birth at home, it is hardly the only reason.

Birth at home often enables the mother to respond more positively to labor. Vermont physician Dr. Thurmond Knight observes, "The quality of labor is often utterly different at home than in a hospital. A woman's strength comes out at a home birth and she welcomes the changes that take place in her body. She is in the most natural place to have a baby—the place where she feels most comfortable and secure. She can make her own decisions rather than submit to protocol. And loved ones surround her— guests in her home—not strangers who control an unfamiliar setting."

There are many advantages to childbirth at home:

♦ *The parents are in complete control.* A central theme common to many home birth parents is the desire to reclaim control over the childbearing experience. In her own home, the mother does not have to relinquish control of her birth experience to medical staff. "One reason I had a home birth is that I wanted to be the one who led the show," recalls one mother, "not have someone else tell me what I could or couldn't do." Many women today want to reassert control over their bodies and their medical care. In the words of California nurse-midwife June Whitson, who helps at both birth center and home births, "By acknowledging that we feel comfortable helping a woman give birth at home, we are telling her that we trust her body and her instincts to do what is best to have her baby in the safest, most comfortable way."

◆ *The mother rarely has to assert herself to get the medical care she wants.* During labor a woman is highly sensitive and vulnerable. It is no time to have to stand up for your rights and fight for the kind of birth you want. "It's your baby, your body," affirms childbirth educator Mariann Martinez of Mystic, Connecticut. "You shouldn't have to fight for what is already yours."

◆ *The mother is free to do whatever she wants during labor.* She is free to eat, drink, get up and walk around, give birth in the position of her choice. She does not have to confront impersonal hospital policies—such as withholding even light meals and liquids from laboring women. She can devote all her attention to her labor. Certified nurse-midwife Alice Bailes attended a birth where the mother moaned, groaned, and grunted quite loudly during labor. Between her contractions, she broke into a big smile and said, "I'm glad I'm home where I can feel comfortable about making these loud sounds without worrying about offending or disturbing anyone." Her six- and two-and-a-half-year-old children started grunting along with their mother when she pushed the baby out into the world.

◆ *The mother can invite whomever she wants to be with her.* Every mother should have the right to share her birth with the person or people of her choice. This is a basic human right not legally recognized. Many hospitals restrict the number of people the mother can have with her during labor. A few don't even allow the father to attend unless he has taken special childbirth classes.

◆ *The health care providers are guests in the mother's home.* Lisa Jensen, licensed New Hampshire midwife, considers this a major difference between home and hospital birth. "The home birth practitioner is a visitor present at the parents' invitation, not an authority who is in charge." Many parents appreciate this distinction. Dr. Howard Marchbanks tells his clients, "I always feel as if I am a guest in your home, whom you have invited to attend the special occasion of your birth."

◆ *The mother can avoid unnecessary medical intervention.* Injudicious intervention, though often routine in hospitals, may cause complications and increase the risk of cesarean section. At home the mother is at a reduced risk of iatrogenic (doctor-caused) medical complications and nosocomial (hospital-caused) infection and other problems in childbearing.

◆ *The risk of infection is reduced for both mother and baby.* During pregnancy the baby receives antibodies from the mother via the placenta. These antibodies provide immunities to familiar family germs, making home-born babies less likely to get such bacterial or viral diseases as urinary tract infection. Hospitals host unfamiliar and sometimes virulent pathogens that are more likely to cause infections in both mother and baby.

◆ *Many mothers feel more comfortable laboring at home.* The hospital is such a clinical environment. At home the mother is on her own familiar turf—the ideal place to begin her family.

◆ *The mother does not have to move from one place to another during labor.* While being up and about can enhance labor's progress, moving from one's home to the hospital may have just the opposite effect and cause labor to slow. When you think about it, moving from one place to another is an odd custom—like moving from one place to another during lovemaking. It can be done, but it's seldom the most comfortable or effective way.

◆ *Parents and baby remain together.* The immediate postpartum period is usually less traumatic for the baby and the mother at home. Parents and infant can enjoy immediate and prolonged bonding time without interruption. Such pediatric procedures as weighing and measuring the baby can wait as long as the parents want and then take place in the presence of family.

◆ *Home is the only place some parents can have the birth experience they want.* If you would like to have siblings attend the birth, the father catch the baby, or a midwife attend the delivery, you may not be able to find a childbearing center or hospital to adapt to your plans.

◆ *Home birth costs a fraction of what a hospital birth costs.* The parents avoid the hospital fee, a significant portion of maternity care cost. This advantage is especially attractive to parents who don't have optimum health insurance.

Yet another advantage of home birth is the special, almost magical beauty that we cannot create in a hospital no matter how comfortable the environment or how positive the staff. In the words of Dr. Thurmond Knight, "Births I've witnessed in parents' homes are the most beautiful and holy I've ever attended. Nothing equals home for peace and privacy. Home is unquestionably the best place for normal labor and birth, providing a woman is healthy."

Interestingly, Dr. Knight was trained in a conventional Florida hospital and, like most American physicians, had never witnessed a home birth. A neighbor invited him to attend her home birth in the role of a friend, not a practitioner, and that birth was the turning point of his career. The home birth was unlike anything he had ever witnessed in a hospital. "The way I had looked at deliveries in the past had no meaning after this home birth," he recalls. "In that holy silence of that farmhouse bedroom, I had seen what childbirth was meant to be."

Despite the many benefits of childbirth at home, there are a few disadvantages to weigh and consider:

◆ Home birth services are not available everywhere. In some areas parents are not able to find a competent home birth practitioner.

◆ The medical establishment does not yet widely accept home birth. The parents who choose home birth risk the disapproval of some health professionals, and even of relatives and friends.

◆ Home birth is limited to the low-risk mother. The mother with medical complications cannot safely give birth at home. It is not possible, even with careful screening, to guarantee that any particular mother is low-risk. Problems can always develop at the last minute that are impossible to predict in advance.

◆ There is no effective way to provide rapid emergency delivery in the home environment. For example, if severe fetal distress arises, requiring an emergency cesarean, the mother must be transported to the hospital immediately. Distance to the hospital and travel conditions should be considered.

◆ Blood transfusions in rare cases of hemorhage cannot be effectively given outside of a hospital.

Should You Give Birth at Home?

Parents from many backgrounds—from farmers to physicians—elect to give birth at home. Should you? The first thing to ask yourself is where you will feel must comfortable. Whether you opt for home, childbearing center, or hospital, you are most likely to labor efficiently if you are comfortable in your birthing environment. Learning as much as you can about each will help you decide which setting seems most congenial.

If home is where you want to be, the next thing to decide is whether home birth is safe for you. Practitioners vary in their criteria for predicting who can give birth at home with relative safety, but most agree that:

◆ The mother should be in good health and at low risk for complications.

◆ She should be attended by a well-trained physician or midwife with adequate medical supplies, including oxygen and resuscitation equipment.

◆ She should be prepared to leave her home and go to the nearest medical facility should complications develop.

◆ Her home should be within a ten- to fifteen-minute drive of a hospital. The mother who lives farther from the hospital may want to consider a childbearing center. Lacking a nearby childbirth center, a few parents have temporarily relocated to a home near a medical facility.

Which Mothers Should Not Plan a Home Birth?

The mother with any of the following is probably safest giving birth in a hospital:

- Diabetes (depending on the severity)
- High blood pressure
- Heart disease
- Kidney disease
- An active case of genital herpes at the time of labor
- Anemia that persists until the time of delivery
- Rh-negative blood with antibody sensitization (a blood incompatibility presenting a risk to the baby)
- Unexplained bleeding during pregnancy
- Preeclampsia (a pregnancy disease characterized by high blood pressure, swelling, and protein in the urine)
- Polyhydramnios or oligohydramnios (too much or too little amniotic fluid)
- Premature labor
- Postmature labor
- Multiple pregnancy
- Baby in the breech position
- History of previous unexplained stillbirth
- History of hemorrhage (Many health care providers will assess the reason for hemorrhage, as this condition is frequently iatrogenic.)
- Any other condition for which hospitalization may be advisable

In addition, you should make sure you have thorough prenatal care. And you may need to arrange for extra help at home after the birth. Take responsibility for planning your birth carefully, and become as well-educated about childbirth as possible.

Since home birth is not yet widely accepted in this country, preparation is often more difficult than preparation for hospital birth. Depending on where your home is, you may have to look harder for a competent health care provider. You will purchase many of your own supplies. In addition, you must locate a backup hospital in case a transfer becomes necessary.

Researchers have surveyed home birth parents. Though a few home birth mothers are uneducated, most do not differ in educational or socioeconomic background from other mothers. Studies have shown that women choosing home birth are more educated about childbirth than others. Most consider their options carefully before making a choice.

As Elizabeth Hosford, CNM, past coordinator of the Maternity Center Association in New York City, observes, "In many ways home birth couples are in the forefront with others who are leading the way toward greater individual responsibility for health. They are keenly interested and highly motivated."

Home birth parents in general have philosophical differences from their hospital birth counterparts. Most view childbirth as a normal, healthy process, respect the value of family bonding and the father's participation, and believe that parents should take personal responsibility for their own and their children's health care. Most home birth parents also breastfeed, a vital health advantage to the newborn.

Home birth requires more preparation than hospital birth. You will need to:

♦ Make the decision

♦ Choose a home-birth health-care provider

♦ Provide for an emergency backup physician (if your health care provider hasn't already arranged for one.)

♦ Choose a backup hospital

♦ Get proper supplies

MAKING THE DECISION

Like many couples, Cheri and Martin didn't begin to investigate their options until Cheri was six months pregnant. Her obstetrician gave offhand responses to many of her questions. Meanwhile, a friend had spoken highly of her own home birth. "We were both unsure about it. I began to read everything I could in the library about childbirth," recalls Cheri. After she and Martin weighed their options, she felt "it was better to have the baby at home."

Another couple, Jean and Tony, who have two sons and two daughters, didn't learn about home birth until after their first daughter was born in a hospital. Jean says, "I didn't have my first child at home because at the time I didn't even realize you could do that! My husband was a little unsure about home birth at first. But after reading and praying about it, we felt home birth was right for us."

Ideally, you and your mate should jointly make the decision. If both parents agree, anxiety and negative feelings in the birth place will be minimized.

Make your choice with care. "Having the baby at home now seems normal and natural to me, but our decision didn't come easily," says Bill, a father of two in east Texas. His wife, Linda, considered a home birth largely to avoid another cesarean section. She recalls, "The more we read, the more we felt certain our chances at being permitted to have a vaginal birth were very slight in our local hospital, which had a cesarean section rate of 25 percent. Once we made the decision, it was like a weight lifted from my shoulders. I felt exuberant about this pregnancy. I was thrilled with the sense of control I regained." (Depending on the type of uterine incision, vaginal birth after a previous cesarean is usually quite safe. If you had a cesarean, check with your physician or midwife to be sure vaginal delivery will be safe for you.)

As more parents learn about home birth, more will choose it. Many are simply unaware of this option. Or they don't realize what home birth offers. For example, Tami Michele, a childbirth educator in Grandville, Michigan, says, "I had the typical American attitude of 'I believe birth is a natural physiological body function, but it's best to have a baby in the hospital in case anything goes wrong.'" Consequently she gave birth to her first two children in the hospital. Then a couple in one of her

> ## Requirements for a Safe Home Birth
>
> The mother who plans to give birth at home should have all of the following:
>
> ◆ Good health
> ◆ Thorough prenatal care
> ◆ Low risk status
> ◆ A well-trained health care provider with adequate medical supplies including oxygen and resuscitation equipment
> ◆ Plans for emergency back-up, transfer to the hospital, and help at home after birth
> ◆ A commitment to become well informed about childbirth.

childbirth classes decided to have a baby at home with a midwife. The parents asked Tami to be their labor support person.

"I was shocked and nervous about it," Tami recalls. But she believed it was a mother's right to give birth in the place where she felt safest. Tami supported the parents during the birth, and the experience altered her feelings. "As I left their home, I had a feeling about this birth that I had never experienced before. Each baby's birth is a miracle, but there was something so special about this one. The midwife had a certain way of handling the birth which I had never seen in an obstetrician or a hospital. The mother worked with the long labor so well. And the baby had a peaceful contentment about him, like he was glad to be here."

Tami's next two children were born at home.

Choosing a Home-Birth Health-Care Provider

Most home birth practitioners are midwives. The renaissance of midwifery in the United States is due partly to the increasing number of parents seeking competent, supportive, home birth health care providers. Many midwives require their clients to have, besides midwifery prenatal care, routine prenatal exams with a physician to screen for possible complications. Most midwives also bring an assistant with them to home births.

Physicians rarely attend home births.

All competent health care providers do regular prenatal exams. These include checking blood pressure, weight gain, blood samples, urine samples, fetal growth, and fetal heart tones. Most home birth practitioners also spend time with clients to give nutritional suggestions, ensure the normalcy of the pregnancy, and discuss concerns and emotional factors with the parents.

The health care provider will probably make at least one prenatal visit to your home to be sure you have adequate supplies. Many will also make a postpartum visit.

The health care provider who attends your birth will do a newborn exam. However, you should also pick out your baby's health care provider for the weeks and months following birth.

Interview the health care provider. A safe home-birth practitioner will meet all of the following requirements:

- *Thorough training and experience.* This is your primary concern. You want to be sure your practitioner can recognize complications and handle an emergency. Most midwives are well trained. Many have better safety statistics than obstetricians. However, a few learn "on the job" without supervision. Don't hesitate to ask questions. How many home births has she attended? (Some have attended fewer than fifty, others several hundred.) How was she trained? Is she licensed by the state or certified? Can she do suturing should you need a laceration repaired? Some midwives have to call someone else to come to the home or transport mothers to the hospital should suturing be required. Ask the practitioner how she handles emergencies.

- *Adequate medical equipment.* Your health care provider should be able to supply a fetoscope or doppler (hand-held ultrasound device that amplifies the fetal heart tones), oxygen for infant resuscitation, appropriate medications such as oxytocic drugs should hemorrhage occur, suturing materials, and other equipment. The practitioner may request that you purchase some supplies.

- *Adequate physician backup.* If you choose a midwife for your primary health care provider, you or the midwife should have arrangements with a physician in case an emergency arises requiring a physician's intervention.

◆ *Backup arrangements with a hospital.* Should a sudden complication require a last-minute transfer, your health care provider should have arrangements to transfer you without delay. Ask what criteria she has for transferring clients to the hospital.

To locate a good home birth practitioner, talk with childbirth educators, midwives, family practitioners, and obstetricians in your area. If the health care provider you contact does not attend home births, ask for a referral. If nothing else, you will make health professionals aware that more parents are requesting home birth services.

Unfortunately, some areas have no physicians who attend home birth or support for the midwives who do. Consequently, you may have difficulty finding a home birth practitioner.

Giving Birth Alone

"I didn't call the midwife soon enough!" recalls Jean, a new mother. "My husband, Tony, ended up catching the baby. When I said, 'The baby's coming!' he ran to the window and shouted, 'Pam's not here yet!'

"'Too late for Pam,' I told him. 'Come sit! I'll tell you what to do.'"

A few parents give birth at home with no professional health care provider present. In Jean and Tony's case, it was an accident, like giving birth on the way to the hospital.

However, some parents plan to give birth without a health care provider, usually for the following reasons:

◆ The parents wish to catch the baby themselves. Some parents choose to be unattended by a professional because they want a father-caught birth. However, parents can also plan for this option more safely with an open-minded health care provider. For example, I caught our second son with a physician present, and our third and fourth sons with a midwife present. Nevertheless, a few families feel this event should not be shared by a professional—particularly a person who is a relative stranger. As one mother put it, "I couldn't bear for anyone besides my husband to touch me."

◆ The parents are unable to create the birth of their choice any other way. In some areas parents cannot find a health care provider who supports their individual plans whether for a father-caught delivery, children at birth, or simply a home birth. David and Lee Stewart's story is a classic example. They were unable to find a midwife or physician to attend the home births of their children, which occurred between 1962 and 1976. Their five healthy children, therefore, were all born without a professional present. (The Stewarts do not suggest that other parents follow their example.) The Stewarts later founded the International Association for Parents and Professionals for Safe Alternatives in Childbirth (NAPSAC), which now has chapters throughout the world. Today NAPSAC publishes books and pamphlets promoting safe, natural birth options. For more information see the Resources section of this book.

◆ The parents feel that birth is a sacred or highly intimate experience to be shared only by the couple or the immediate family. As one mother put it, "We simply felt that birth is a holy event and should be kept in the family if the pregnancy is normal and the baby is healthy."

Do-it-yourself home birth is in part the result of our society's failure to meet the parents' needs for the birth of their choice. The Association for Childbirth at Home, International (ACHI) conducted a research study on do-it-yourself (DIY) home birth. Its founder and president, Tonya Brooks, reports, "We found most DIY couples in southern California were educated people who have the money for and the availability of birth attendants. Their reasons for deliberately choosing a DIY were various. Many had been rudely denied care and had thus become radicalized against all health care providers." Most home birth advocates agree that unattended birth poses a significant risk. Most parents who choose an unattended home birth have no way of monitoring fetal well-being and no way of handling emergencies should they arise. *The Journal of the American Medical Association* published a study conducted by the federal government's Centers for Disease Control of home births that took place in North Carolina between 1974 and 1976. Neonatal mortality rates were 3 per thousand for planned lay midwife–attended home births, 30 per thousand for planned home births with no attendant, and 120 per thousand, for unplanned home births. (By comparison, the neonatal death rate among hospital births was 12 per thousand which included high-risk pregnancies and low-birth-weight babies. Excluding the low-birth-weight babies, the hospital neonatal death rate was 7 per thousand.[6])

Most parents who plan a do-it-yourself birth are aware of the risk. As one mother explains, "We felt unattended home births were more dangerous than attended ones, but the only doctor doing home birth in our area wasn't competent or a man we could talk with. And I was thrown out of my previous OB's office because of my 'nonsensical ideas' about birth. After that, I read books, got a medical textbook, and we decided to do it ourselves."

Another mother says, "I felt the hospital procedures were just as dangerous as an unattended home birth."

Parents who want a do-it-yourself birth should have a competent health professional present only to intervene if necessary. For example, Alice Bailes, CNM, tells the story of one of her favorite "unattended" births:

When I arrived at the parents' home, the parents-to-be were working together in labor. I came into the darkened bedroom quietly and took my place in a corner on the rug. I sat there silently. Then I stood up and said, "Excuse me, I'd like to listen to the baby." After checking the fetal heart tones, I resumed my post in the corner. I remained there for the next hour and a half with brief sorties to the baby to hear the heart tones every twenty minutes or so.

Then the mom moved up onto her side in the bed, where her husband helped her get supported with some pillows. I took my birth set out of my bag, put my instruments in the placenta bowl, put on my gloves, and sat in a corner of the bed where I could see well. The dad sat in front of his wife while she put her knee on his shoulder.

The mom pushed and panted, gently giving counterpressure with one hand to the baby's head, helping it out slowly herself, with her eyes closed. The baby rotated to face her daddy, and he and his wife lifted the baby out and into the mother's arms. It was a beautiful birth, one where the parents did it all.

Many times our mere presence, and only our presence, is all that is necessary. It gives the client the confidence she needs. She may need a health care provider to intervene only if there is a threat to the mother's or the baby's safety. Having a professional present, she can count on our special lifeguard skills.

Choosing a Backup Hospital

A backup hospital within a twenty-minute drive of your home is an essential requirement for a safe home birth. Should a medical emergency arise during labor or the early postpartum period, you may need to transfer to the hospital without delay.

Select your backup hospital during pregnancy. (Choosing a hospital is discussed in chapter 7.) Your health care provider will probably already have arrangements with one or more institutions in the area.

Cheri and Martin chose two backup hospitals, both about the same distance from their home. "We decided if there was a problem during labor to go to the hospital that had a reputation for progressive obstetric care. If there was a problem with the baby, we planned to go to the high-risk center."

If possible, select a hospital that will support your plans. The staff will be far more helpful if a last-minute transfer is necessary.

In many areas of the United States, your choice will be limited. You may not find a hospital with supportive staff and may have to make do with what is available. Unfortunately, planning a safe home birth in America sometimes entails making compromises.

WHEN IS A TRANSFER NECESSARY?

Home birth parents may transfer to the hospital for a variety of reasons. Such life-threatening complications as severe fetal distress, prolapsed cord, or maternal hemorrhage are comparatively rare, but they do sometimes occur. When they do, emergency transfer is mandatory.

More often than not, however, parents transfer for less severe complications. For example, the most common medical problems in more than thirty-five hundred Arizona home birth mothers were premature rupture of membranes, premature labor, and labor delayed beyond forty-two weeks' gestation. In cases like this, there is usually no rush. You can go to the hospital at your leisure.

Whatever the reason, transfer will be less traumatic if you carefully plan for it in advance. Kathleen, a mother who spent much time planning her home birth, recalls, "In my mind, I imagined everything that could go wrong and decided how I wanted each possibility handled. For example, if I had to be transported to a hospital after birth, I had arranged for a healthy breastfeeding friend to come and nurse my baby while I was away. By the time of birth, my husband and midwife knew extensively all my concerns and how I wanted to handle possible problems."

The possibility of transfer is a good reason to draw up a birth options plan (discussed in chapter 3), expressing your preferences for care during labor, birth, and the early postpartum period.

Following are some major reasons mothers transfer from home to hospital. A competent health care provider must diagnose these conditions.

Emergencies

- ◆ *Prolapsed cord.* The umbilical cord precedes the baby's head in the birth canal. This presents a grave danger of fetal asphyxiation and death.
- ◆ *Bright red bleeding during pregnancy or labor.* This is a possible sign that the placenta is overlying the cervix or had detached from the uterine wall. There is a serious danger of fetal death and maternal hemorrhage.
- ◆ *Baby is blue, limp, and not breathing.* This presents a danger of fetal asphyxiation and death, and immediate resuscita-

tion at home is imperative. However, the baby is usually then transferred for further care.

◆ *Fetal heart rate low (under 100) or racing (180).* Known as fetal distress, this presents the danger of inadequate oxygen, brain damage, and death.

◆ *Maternal hemorrhage after birth.* This may be profuse bleeding or a continuous trickle of blood.

Other Reasons for Transfer

◆ *Prolonged rupture of membranes.* There is a risk of infection after twenty-four hours. The health care provider may, however, prefer keeping the mother at home and monitoring for signs of infection.

◆ *Premature labor.* Labor is premature if it begins three weeks or more before the due date.

◆ *Postmature labor.* Labor is postmature if it begins more than three weeks past the due date.

◆ *Greenish or brownish amniotic fluid.* This shows that the baby has passed meconium and may or may not have continued fetal distress. (Meconium is the sticky greenish black substance of the baby's first stool. It sometimes passes in the uterus when the baby is distressed).

◆ *Prolonged labor or lack of progress.* Before transferring to the hospital, try other methods to induce or enhance labor *with your health care provider's approval.* These include walking, lovemaking, nipple stimulation, and relaxation. (Both lovemaking with orgasm and nipple stimulation release the hormone oxytocin, which can trigger labor contractions if the cervix is ripe and the mother is ready to go into labor. This is a more natural and enjoyable way to enhance labor than taking an oxytocic drug.)

◆ *The mother feels that she should be in a hospital.* You may have an intuition that you need medical care in the hospital or that something isn't right. Pay attention to this intuition. Let your body be your guide. If you are more comfortable in a hospital, giving birth there will be a more positive experience.

◆ *Breech position.* In this position the baby's feet or buttocks—rather than head—are first in the birth canal. This is usually, but not always, diagnosed prenatally.

◆ *More than one baby (twins, triplets, or more)*. This is usually, but not always, diagnosed prenatally. Risk increases with the number of babies.

◆ *Placenta does not deliver* within a half hour to an hour after birth.

◆ *Retained placental fragments*. Sometimes not all of the placenta is delivered. A health care provider should remove the retained fragments in the hospital.

◆ *Maternal tears* that the health care provider is unable to repair at home.

◆ *Any other condition* requiring medical treatment or observation.

Home Birth Supplies

Did you ever wonder what all that boiling water in movie and television birth scenes was for? Most often it was for sterilizing scissors, cord clamps, or string to tie the umbilical cord. However, in all the home births I've attended, the only thing I've ever seen people boil water for is tea or coffee.

You will need several things other than boiling water. Check the list that follows and then find out what your health care provider plans to bring and what you should purchase. You can obtain supplies from many drugstores, medical supply houses, or a mail-order business specializing in childbirth supplies.

For Labor and Birth

◆ Two sets of clean sheets, one for birth, one for afterward
◆ A waterproof pad or sheet to prevent staining the mattress (a shower curtain or large plastic tablecloth works fine)
◆ Disposable absorbent pads (such as Chux by Johnson & Johnson or large diapers) to place beneath the mother
◆ Clean towels
◆ Clean washcloths for compresses

- 1–2 dozen sterile gauze pads (for perineal support as the baby is born)
- 6–12 pairs of disposable sterile gloves
- Trash bags
- Oil for massage (unopened vitamin E oil or olive oil is often recommended)
- Umbilical cord clamps
- 3 oz. bulb syringe (to suction mucus from baby's mouth and nose)
- Hot tea and honey and plenty of other liquids
- Food for those attending the birth
- A mirror so the mother can watch the birth
- A large bowl to catch the placenta

For After the Birth

- Cotton balls and rubbing alcohol to cleanse the umbilical cord after it is cut
- Receiving blankets for the newborn

Why the Bias Against Home Birth?

In some children's books or magazines you'll find drawings that include an absurd element such as a dinosaur playing the flute. The object for the child is to pick out what's out of place. Being a consumer of obstetric care in America is a little like that: we must pick out the absurdities. And it's quite a task. There are probably more flute-playing dinosaurs in American childbirth than in the birth customs of just about any other nation in the world.

Throughout anthropological literature you'll find few things stranger than routines associated with typical American birth—from perineal shaving to maternal-infant separation during the first hour after birth. Since we are so used to such things, we often fail to see how absurd they are.

One of the strangest things about American birth is the widespread prejudice against home birth. In the Netherlands, a country with a much lower infant mortality rate than ours, half of all births take place at home. Until the 1930s the overwhelming majority of births in this country occurred at home. Suddenly having a baby at home is considered unconventional behavior. As one home birth practitioner puts it, "It is a comment on our times that we, who want childbirth to again become an intimate family affair filled with the security of one's home and the love of one's family, are considered radicals."

Once during a workshop for childbirth professionals, I briefly mentioned home birth twice in seven hours. A nurse wrote a note on her evaluation form stating that she was against parents who gave birth at home because she had heard of complications developing. One might turn the tables. A host of health problems often result from the hospital and obstetrical routines.

Often parents suffer from the prejudice against home birth. As childbirth educator and anthropologist Lester Hazell observes, "If you have your baby at home, you will be going counter to the social trend. This means that you have to brace yourself against remarks if you tell people ahead of time you plan to do this. It also means that if anything goes wrong, you are in a position of having brought it on yourself and your baby. Our strange society will not hold it against you if your baby is palsied or his intelligence is stunted by too much anesthesia in the hospital, but if he is born at home with a birthmark or a clubfoot, the fault will be called yours!"

Home birth parents also face the harassment of health professionals. Some doctors, for example, refer to home birth as "child abuse"—a statement as foolish as it is heinous. And there are some physicians who even refuse to provide prenatal care to a mother who intends to give birth at home with a midwife. (In my opinion, this is a form of malpractice far graver than those for which physicians are usually sued.) Any physician who refuses to provide a mother quality prenatal care because he doesn't agree with her choice of birth place is hardly concerned with healthy mothers and babies! There also are unfortunate cases of home birth mothers who transfer to hospitals because of complications and meet gross insensitivity. For example, one Florida mother had a retained placenta, a complication having nothing to do with the place of birth. She transferred from home to hospital. During her hospital stay, several nurses criticized her decision to give birth at home with comments like, "You must have been crazy to attempt a home birth!"

Fortunately, many health professionals who disagree with parents' choices recognize that they have the right to choose.

Researchers Deborah A. Sullivan and Rose Weitz surveyed physicians throughout Arizona. They found something almost impossible to believe. Despite the excellent outcomes of licensed lay midwives, three-quarters of the obstetricians and two-thirds of the family physicians wanted the state to outlaw home births with licensed lay midwives. Many wanted to deny obstetricians the right to attend births at home as well.

. Why do some physicians oppose home birth? Many feel it represents a giant step backward. Home birth frightens many physicians, midwives, and nurses who have been constantly surrounded by complications, some stemming from poor maternal health, others from obstetrical procedures. The daily confrontation with problems in the hospital reinforces the belief that birth is fraught with risks. Accordingly, the practitioner develops a hesitancy or fear of being away from technical equipment and staff that can help in emergencies. By contrast, home birth practitioners see primarily normal births and learn to deal with complications such as umbilical cord prolapse by transferring the mother to a hospital. Their view that home birth is safe is continually reinforced.

Economy is another reason behind the opposition. Home birth is less profitable for the practitioner, who may be in a laboring woman's home for hours. While in the hospital, the physician can take care of other responsibilities, see other patients, even provide care for several mothers at once. While this makes perfect sense to the physician, there is no reason it should influence your choice.

Concern about malpractice also looms large in physician resistance to home birth. As one physician puts it, "I would be more supportive of lay midwives if my malpractice insurance wasn't twenty-three thousand dollars." It is easy to understand his feeling. Today, in our suit-happy society, it is a risk to be a conventional obstetrician, let alone one who bucks the established patterns of practice. The health care consumer is largely to blame for the malpractice crisis because of the high numbers of unwarranted suits. We might consider that while obstetricians are frequently sued, rarely is a suit brought against a midwife. This could be partly because the midwife makes every effort to help the mother give birth the way she wants.

Another factor contributing to health professionals' resistance is a stubborn refusal to consider something beyond their immediate experience. As researchers Sullivan and Weitz observe, "Physicians may present appropriate evidence to bolster their opposition or may choose to ignore evidence that contradicts their preconceived ideas."[7] They point out that physicians ignore home birth studies as they have ignored evidence in favor of such other health care alternatives as acupuncture.

Looking Ahead

Planned childbirth at home with a midwife, physician, or physician-midwife team is the alternative of choice for an increasing number of parents. Home unquestionably provides a more comfortable, more positive birth environment for many parents. Studies to date have provided favorable information about childbirth at home. It is my hope that more extensive studies will follow.

As more parents elect to give birth at home, home birth services will become more widely available. Home birth will also become safer. Safety for mother and child is greatly improving as more health professional teams with emergency backup are more widely distributed and more hospitals are willing to adapt to the needs of parents in their community who choose to give birth at home. For now, home birth parents are still pioneers; they must still oppose the system. It takes courage to stand up against well-established medical policies (even when the policies rest on prejudice rather than science) and to act on one's beliefs. Some home birth parents become champions for change, inspiring others to follow their example.

The parents who give birth at home today are blazing the way for a safer, saner obstetrics when the time comes for our children to give birth their way.

For Us to Create

In many ways we are emerging from an obstetrical dark age. Healthy, rewarding options for mother and baby are slowly replacing the dehumanizing maternity care of the past. As more parents carefully plan their births; select their hospitals; interview their health care providers, making a change of provider when they are not satisfied; and become actively involved in all aspects of their maternity care, the face of childbirth in America will change.

For now there is much to be improved. Many changes are yet to be made. For example, home birth services are not available everywhere, and in many childbearing centers, screening requirements are still overly rigid, preventing hundreds of healthy mothers from giving birth within their doors. Although hospitals are improving, institutions with all the ideal characteristics described in the chapter about hospital birth are rare. In many areas certified nurse-midwives still don't have hospital privileges, and direct-entry midwives do not yet have hospital privileges anywhere. Many nurse-midwives and physicians still will not attend home births. And unless they live close to one of the very few centers in the world where waterbirth is available, most parents must go to great lengths to prepare for this option.

Conventional medical practice has had a virtual monopoly on health care since the 1800s. Today this situation is changing. People are beginning to realize that other methods of health care, including homeopathy, chiropractic medicine, and acupuncture, are safe and effective. The changing face of childbirth cannot be separated from the widespread trend toward recognizing other

226

methods of health care. Eventually the view that labor is a normal, natural event—a celebration, not an illness—will replace traditional views of labor.

Yet many birth options are still in their newborn stages. If they are to grow and survive, dramatic changes must be made in the way many professionals view childbirth. As David Stewart of NAPSAC points out, the current maternal-child health care system is seriously flawed. It cannot simply be modified but needs fundamental changes.

First, we need to adopt a new model of childbirth that encompasses the laboring mother's psychological, emotional, and behavioral as well as physiological changes. All health professionals should know this model. The hundreds of nurses and midwives who attend the mind-over-labor workshop teach others, including residents and physicians, about the laboring mind response, helping them to understand the experience of labor in addition to childbirth's anatomy and physiology. Frequently I get calls from physicians who, having learned about the laboring mind response, feel they understand labor for the first time. Then comes the frustrating question: "Why don't they teach us this in medical school?" Indeed, why?

Second, we need major changes in legislation, granting parents freedom of choice in childbirth. This means allowing direct-entry midwives as well as certified nurse-midwives to practice throughout the United States without hiding their practice from legal persecution like Christians in the catacombs. The major medical organizations also need some sort of legislation forbidding hospitals and other physicians from punishing a practitioner because he or she attends a home birth. Parents do not have the freedom to choose childbirth options when practitioners who attend home births are threatened with denial of privileges.

Third, we need many more publicized studies. Research has proven without question that childbirth companions improve health outcomes for mothers and babies. Of course, there are a few closed-minded individuals who resist this option. However, most childbirth practitioners recognize and accept these new health professionals. Other major areas requiring more research are home birth, direct-entry midwifery care, childbearing center birth, and waterbirth. Thousands of health professionals remain ignorant of the impressive safety statistics associated with these options. Those who are familiar with the laboring mind response realize that an emotionally positive environment leads to a more efficient labor. This is common sense. However, to effect even greater change than we are witnessing today, we need to prove it statistically. We also need to measure the effects of guided imagery on the mother's experience of labor and prove with research what health professionals who have used the method know from experience: that guided imagery reduces fear, pain, the length of labor, and the likelihood of a cesarean.

What You Can Do

You can help shape the future of childbirth. Readers who are alarmed that one in every four American mothers gives birth by cesarean surgery, who are horrified by unfair laws discriminating against midwifery care, or who are disappointed about the lack of options for birth methods in their area can work toward change. Many expectant and new parents become childbirth activists working for change in their community.

If you would like to see more childbirth options available in your area, you can take several steps:

- ◆ *Apply consumer pressure.* Pressure from consumers triggers change, particularly in hospitals. If you are dissatisfied with the hospitals in your area, write to hospital administrators and let them know why you will not (or did not) give birth in that institution. Do not patronize a hospital that doesn't offer humanized maternity care. If you have had a disappointing birth experience in the hospital, let administrators know about it. If enough people express dissatisfaction with rigid policies, lack of midwifery services, inadequate backup for home birth services, and overly interventive obstetrical care, changes will occur.
- ◆ *Set up educational programs for parents and health professionals.* Invite a health professional to plan a workshop educating parents and professionals about their options in your area. Education alone is sometimes enough to trigger major breakthroughs. In addition, planning a workshop can give you effective local publicity. By generating radio,

TV, and newspaper publicity for the birth method of your choice, you make other health care consumers aware of their choices.

◆ *Organize a childbirth group.* A group of parents and professionals working together can educate health care consumers, disseminate information about birth options, provide support for VBAC mothers and others with special needs, and lobby for legislative change in midwifery laws. Don't understimate the power of a small group. La Leche League International, an organization with millions of members worldwide supporting breast-feeding mothers, began with seven women who wanted to offer support to others. The Association of Childbirth Companions will help you get your own group started.

◆ *Get publicity for birth methods not currently available in your area.* Present information on the safety and benefits of a particular childbirth option at public health meetings, before the board of trustees at publicly funded hospitals, at hospital childbirth classes, health fairs, conferences, and any other meeting or organization associated with childbirth.

◆ *Take responsibility for your own birth.* This is the single most important step to take in inspiring change. I often hear mothers make remarks like "The physician allowed my husband to catch the baby," or "The hospital allowed my mother to remain with us during the birth." Such statements reflect how far the mother is from seeing herself as a paying consumer in charge of the show. Remember it's *your* birth and *your* baby, not the nurse's, the midwife's, the physician's, or the hospital's. Your health care provider is someone you hire. Taking responsibility for your own birth increases the likelihood you'll have a rewarding, fulfilling, and healthy birth.

Many believe that physicians are responsible for shaping the future of childbirth, as they are the ones who design the procedures. Others believe that hospitals, who write the policies, are responsible. Some look to legislators, who make the laws.

But the future of childbirth does not lie with any of these people. It is we, the parents, who will determine the changes that will be made. Ultimately, childbirth reflects our relationship with nature, our feelings about our bodies, our attitudes about sexuality, and our beliefs about birth. We shape our own birth experiences by what we believe about birth and by the choices we make.

The future of childbirth is for us to create.

Appendix

Creating a Class Curriculum

Most childbirth educators today teach the *Mind Over Labor* method. However, a few instructors neglect to cover vital information you should have to prepare for labor including: *the laboring mind response*, which gives both parents necessary insight into the experience of labor (not just labor's anatomy and physiology), the method of using guided imagery in pregnancy and labor (the basis of the *Mind Over Labor* method), the *pros and cons* of obstetrical routines and intervention, and how to draw up a personalized *birth options plan*. If your educator does not cover these items, it is often better either to educate yourself or supplement your education with your own curriculum. Bear in mind, a class that offers inadequate information or that is designed to make you a compliant patient can do far more harm than good.

The following information is from *The Mind Over Labor Manual for Childbirth Professionals* and is designed to be handed out in childbirth classes, prenatal appointments, and elsewhere.

It is a sample six-week curriculum to help parents prepare for labor. You can combine guided imagery with breathing patterns, but if you follow this curriculum, you'll find you probably won't need to do so. All of the guided imagery exercises in this curriculum are described in the book *Mind Over Labor*. (If the book is not in your bookstore, ask the manager to order it for you. Or you can order it yourself by calling toll-free 800-557-2229.)

Start this curriculum at any time during pregnancy.

Week 1

- Read the book *Mind Over Labor*. (Spend several weeks on this if you prefer.)
- Learn and practice *Autogenic Stress Release*.
- Learn and practice *The Special Place*.

Week 2

- Learn about all your options regarding medical procedures and obstetrical routines.
- Practice *Autogenic Stress Release*.
- Practice *The Special Place* and use affirmations or practice goal achievement in the form of visualizing the desired outcome regarding your birth (such as imaging yourself handling contractions smoothly).

Week 3

- Create a written birth plan, being specific about all medical interventions and obstetrical procedures.
- Learn and practice *The Radiant Breath* and *Getting in Touch With the Unborn Child*

Week 4

- Practice *Autogenic Stress Release*.
- Practice *The Special Place*.
- Learn about tapping your inner resources by asking your inner self a question while in *The Special Place*.
- Evaluate your choice of both health care provider and birth setting and make last minute changes if appropriate.

Week 5

- Practice *The Special Place.*
- Learn and practice *The Mountain Hike.*

Week 6

- Go over all the exercises you have learned
- Learn additional exercises to be used *only* during labor, including *The Opening Flower, Imagining the Birth,* and *The Rainbow.* Do not practice these during pregnancy but be sure both you and your birth partner have them nearly committed to memory so you can recall them or your partner can recall them during labor. *Do not wait until the last minute to do this!*

Notes

Chapter 1

1. Wagner, Marsden, G., "Infant Mortality in Europe: Implications for the United States," *Journal of Public Health Policy* 88 (Winter): 473–84.

2. Hosford, Elizabeth, "The Home Birth Movement," *Journal of Nurse-Midwifery* 21, no. 3 (Fall 1978): 29–30.

Chapter 2

1. Newton, Niles. *Maternal Emotions* (New York: Paul B. Hoeber, 1982).

2. Sidenbladh, Eric. *Water Babies* (New York: St. Martin's Press, 1982), 92.

3. Odent, Michael. *Birth Reborn* (New York: Pantheon Books, 1984), 74.

4. Ibid., 80.

5. Rosenthal, Michael. *Pre- and Perinatal Psychology News* 2, no. 1 (Spring, 1988): 20.

6. Church, Linda. *Journal of Nurse-Midwifery* 34, no. 4 (July/August 1989): 166.

7. Rivers, Anne. *Waterbirth* (Hawaii: self-published, 1984) 11.

8. Kennell, John, et al., "Continuous Emotional Support During Labor in a U.S. Hospital," *Journal of the American Medical Association*, 265, no. 17 (May 1991): 2197–2201.

Chapter 3

1. Sagov, Stanley, et al. *Home Birth: A Practitioner's Guide to Birth Outside the Hospital* (Rockland, Md.: Aspen Systems Corp., 1984), 23.

2. Newton, Niles, "The Effect of Fear and Disturbance In Labor," in *Twenty-first Century Obstetrics Now*, ed. Stewart & Stewart (Marble Hill, Mo.: NAPSAC Publications, 1977): 62–71.

Chapter 4

1. Wagner, Marsden, "The Dutch System of Home Birth," in *Twenty-first Century Obstetrics Now*, ed. Stewart & Stewart (Marble Hill, Mo: NAPSAC Publications, 1977): 289.

2. Kloosterman, G. J. ibid., iii.

235

3. Kantor, H. et al., "Value of Shaving the Pudendal-Perineal Area in Delivery Preparation," *Obstetrics and Gynecology* 25 (1965): 509–12.

4. Lynaugh, Kathleen H., "The Effects of Early Elective Amniotomy on the Length of Labor and the Condition of the Fetus," *Journal of Nurse-Midwifery* 25 (1980): 3–9.

5. Kubli, F., "Influence of Labor on Fetal Acid-Base Balance," *Clinical Obstetrics and Gynecology* 11 (1968): 168–191, and C. Wood, "Transient Fetal Acidosis and Artificial Rupture of the Membranes," *Australia–New Zealand Journal of Obstetrics and Gynecology* 11 (1971): 221–25.

6. Friedman, E. and M. Sachtelben, "Amniotomy and the Course of Labor," *Obstetrics and Gynecology* 22 (1963): 755–70.

7. Caldeyro-Barcia, R., et al., "Adverse Perinatal Effects of Early Amniotomy During Labor," *Modern Perinatal Medicine*, ed. L. Gluck (Chicago: Year Book Medical Publishers, 1974).

8. National Institutes of Health, *Antenatal Diagnostics*, publication no. 79-1973, Bethesda, Md. (April 1979): 344.

9. Kelso, I., "An Assessment of Continuous Fetal Heart Rate Monitoring in High-Risk Pregnancy," *American Journal of Obstetrics and Gynecology* 131, no. 5 (1978): 526–32, and Haverkamp, A., et al., "The Evaluation of Continuous Fetal Heart Rate Monitoring in High-Risk Pregnancy, *American Journal of Obstetrics and Gynecology* 1, no. 3 (June 1976): 125.

10. Stewart & Stewart, ed., "Do We Really Need Monitors?" in *Compulsory Hospitalization*, (Marble Hill, Mo.: NAPSAC Publications 1979): 137.

11. Minkoff, H., and R. Schwartz, "The Rising Cesarean Section Rate: Can It Safely Be Reversed?" *Obstetrics and Gynecology* 56, no. 2 (August 1980): 59.

12. Shy, Kirkwood K., et al., "Effects of Electronic Fetal-Heart-Rate Monitoring," *New England Journal of Medicine* (March 1, 1990).

13. Liu, Y., "Position During Labor and Delivery: History and Perspective," *Journal of Nurse-Midwifery* 24, no. 3 (May/June 1979).

14. Caldeyro-Barcia, Roberto, "Supine Called Worst Position During Labor and Delivery," *Obstetrics and Gynecology News* (June 1975).

15. Naroll F., et al., "Position of Women in Childbirth: A Study in Data Quality Control," *American Journal of Obstetrics and Gynecology* 82 (1961): 943–54.

16. Russell, J., "The Rationale of Primitive Delivery Positions," *British Journal of Obstetrics and Gynecology* 89 (1982): 712–15, and Roberts, Joyce, "Alternative Positions for Childbirth, Part I: First Stage of Labor," and "Part II: Second Stage of Labor," *Journal of Nurse-Midwifery* 25 (1980): 11–30.

17. Caire, J., "Are Current Rates of Cesarean Justified?" *Southern Medical Journal* 71, no. 5 (May 1978): 18.

18. Family Birth Center, current statistics from January 22, 1979, through December 31, 1989, Providence Hospital, Southfield, Mich.

19. Calder, A. A., et al., "Increased Bilirubin Levels in Neonates After Induction of Labor by Intravenous Prostaglandin or Oxytocin," *Lancet* 2 (1974): 1339–1342, and Oski, F.A., "Oxytocin and Hyperbilirubinemia," *American Journal of Disabled Child* 129 (1975): 1139–1140.

20. Banta, David, and Stephen Thacker, "The Risks and Benefits of Episiotomies: A Review," *Birth* 9 (1982): 25–30.

21. Barnet, C. R., et al., "Neonatal Side of Inter-actional Deprivation," *Pediatrics* 54 (1970): 197, and Klaus, M. H. and J. H. Kennel, *Maternal-Infant Bonding: The Impact of Early Separation or Loss on Family Development* (St. Louis: C. V. Mosby, 1976).

22. McBride, A., "Compulsory Rooming-in in the Ward and Private Newborn Service at Duke Hospital," *Journal of the American Medical Association* 145 (1951), 625.

23. Klaus, Marshall H., and John H. Kennel, "Mothers Separated From Their Newborn Infants," *Pediatric Clinics of North America* 17 (1970): 1016–1037.

24. Peterson, G., unpublished manuscript cited in *Twenty-first Century Obstetrics Now* (Marble Hill: NAPSAC Publications, 1977), 179.

25. Klaus, Marshall H., and John H. Kennell. *Maternal-Infant Bonding*

26. Varney, Helen. *Nurse-Midwifery* (Boston: Blackwell Scientific Publications, 1980), 353.

27. MacFarlane, Aidan. *The Psychology of Childbirth* (Cambridge, Mass.: Harvard University Press, 1978): 69.

Chapter 5

1. National Institutes of Health, *Antenatal Diagnostics*, no. 79-1973, Bethesda, Md., (April 1979).

2. Minkoff, H., and R. Schwartz, "The Rising Cesarean Section Rate: Can It Safely Be Reversed?" *Obstetrics and Gynecology*, 56, no. 2 (August 1980)

3. Paul, R., et al., "Clinical Fetal Monitoring: Its Effect on Cesarean Section Rate and Perinatal Mortality: Five-Year Trends," *Postgraduate Medicine* 61 (1977): 160, and Caire, J., "Are Current Rates of Cesarean Justified?" *Southern Medical Journal* 71, no. 5 (May 1978)

4 Paul, R., et al., "Clinical Fetal Monitoring."

Chapter 6

1. Wertz, Richard, and Dorothy Wertz. *Lying-in: A History of Childbirth in America* (New York: Schocken Books, 1979), 119–24.

2. Rooks, Judith, and J. Eugene Haas. *Nurse-Midwifery in America* (American College of Nurse-Midwives Foundation, 1986), 116.

3. Wagner, Marsden G., "Infant Mortality in Europe: Implications for the United States," *Journal of Public Health Policy* 88 (Winter): 473–84.

4. Stewart, David. *The Five Standards for Safe Childbearing* (Marble Hill, Mo.: NAPSAC Reproductions, 1981), 112.

5. Sullivan, Deborah A., and Rose Weitz. *Labor Pains: Modern Midwives and Home Birth* (New Haven: Yale University Press, 1988).

6. Gaskin, Ina May. *Spiritual Midwifery* (Summertown, Tenn.: The Book Publishing Company), 474–75.

7. Ibid., 122–123.

8. Montgomery, T., "A Case for Nurse-Midwives," *American Journal of Obstetrics and Gynecology* 109: 50–58.

9. Institute of Medicine, "Prenatal Care: Reaching Mothers, Reaching Infants," ed. Sara S. Brown (Washington, D.C.: National Academy Press, 1988).

10. Mehl, L., "Research on Alternatives: What It Tells Us About Hospitals," in *Twenty-first Century Obstetrics Now*, Vol. 2, ed. Stewart & Stewart, (Marble Hill, Mo.: NAPSAC International, 1985, 171–207.

11. Boyer, Ernest L. *Midwifery in America: A Profession Reaffirmed* (The Carnegie Foundation, 1990), 1.

12. Wertz, Richard W. *Lying-in: A History of Childbirth in America* (New York: Schocken Books, 1979), 119–124.

13. Stewart, David. *The Five Standards For Safe Childbearing* (Marble Hill, Mo.: NAPSAC Reproductions, 1981), 112.

Chapter 7

1. Faison, J.B., et al., "The Childbearing Center: An Alternative Birth Setting," *Obstetrics and Gynecology* 54, no. 4 (October 1979).

2. McKay, Susan, and Celeste R. Phillips. *Family Centered Maternity Care* (Rockville, Md.: Aspen Systems Corporation, 1984), 101.

3. Waryas, F. S., and M.B. Luebbers, "A Cluster System for Maternity Care, *Maternal Child Nursing* 2 (March/April 1986): 98–100.

4. DeVries, R., "Image and Reality: An Evaluation of Hospital Alternative Birth Centers," *Journal of Nurse-Midwifery* 28 (1983): 3–39.

5. Kennell, J.H., "The Physiologic Effects of a Supportive Compan-

ion (Doula) During Labor," in *Birth, Interaction, and Attachment* (Silkman, N.J.: Johnson and Johnson, 1982).

Chapter 8

1. Lubic, R. W., "The Rise of the Birth Center Alternative," *The Nation's Health* 7.

2. Eakins, Pamela, *Women and Health* 9, no. 4 (Winter 1984): 35

3. Taffel, S., "Maternal Weight Gain and the Outcome of Pregnancy, United States, 1980," *National Center For Health Statistics and Vital Health Series* 21, no. 44 DHHS publication no. 86–1922. Public Health Service (Washington D.C.: U.S. Government Printing Office, 1986): 9.

4. Daniels, S., *Birth and the Family Journal* 6, no. 4 (Winter 1979): 259–266.

5. Sculphome, A., et al., "A Birth Center Affiliated With the Tertiary Care Center: Comparison of Outcome," *Obstetrics and Gynecology* 67, no. 4 (April l986): 598–603

Chapter 9

1. Mehl, Lewis, et al., "Evaluation of Outcomes of Non-Nurse Midwives: Matched Comparisons With Physicians." *Women and Health* 5 (1980): 17–29.

2. Ibid., 17–29.

3. Sullivan, Deborah A., and Rose Weitz. *Labor Pains: Modern Midwives and Home Birth* (New Haven: Yale University, 1988), 163.

4. "Health Department Data Shows Danger of Home Births," in *American Journal of Obstetricians and Gynecologists*, January 4, 1978.

5. Sagov, Stanley, et al. *Home Birth: A Practitioner's Guide to Birth Outside the Hospital* (Rockland, Md.: Aspen Systems Corp., 1984).

6. Burnett, Claude, A. et al., "Home Delivery and Neonatal Mortality in North Carolina," *Journal of the American Medical Association* 224, no. 24: 2741–2745.

7. Sullivan and Weitz. *Labor Pains*, 31.

Resources

One of your most readily available resources for information is the electronic world-wide *Birth Forum* which anyone can access with a computer and modem. To find the phone number to connect with the *Birth Forum* nearest your home, contact the *Birth Forum* hotline toll-free at (800) 605-0081.

Alternatives in Childbirth

International Association of Parents and Professionals for Safe Alternatives in Childbirth (NAPSAC)
Route 1, Box 646
Marble Hill, Missouri 63764
(314) 238-2010

Birth Defects

Association of Birth Defect Children
Orlando Executive Park
5400 Diplomat Circle, Suite 270
Orlando, Florida 32810
(407) 629-1466

March of Dimes Birth Defects Foundation
1275 Mamaroneck Avenue
White Plains, New York 10605
(914) 428-7100

National Network to Prevent Birth Defects
Box 15309, SE Station
Washington, D.C. 20003
(202) 543-5450

Blind and Visually Impaired

American Council of the Blind
1155 15th Street NW, Suite 720
Washington, D.C. 20005
(202) 393-3666
(800) 424-8666

American Foundation for the Blind
15 West 16th Street
New York, New York 10011
(212) 620-2147
(800) 232-5463

Blind Children's Center
4120 Marathon Street
Box 29159
Los Angeles, California 90029-0159
(213) 664-2153
(800) 222-3566

National Association for Parents of the Visually Impaired
2180 Linway Drive
Beloit, Wisconsin 53511
(608) 362-4945
(800) 562-6265

National Society to Prevent Blindness
500 East Remington Road
Schaumburg, Illinois 60173
(708) 843-2020
(800) 221-3004

Breastfeeding

La Leche League International (LLLI)
9616 Minneapolis Avenue
Franklin Park, Illinois 60131
(708) 455-7730
(800) 525-3243 (800) LA LECHE

Many smaller groups support nursing parents. Some childbirth education organizations have their own nursing mothers' counselors. Local childbirth educators, childbearing centers, and some maternity hospitals may be able to give you local referrals.

Cesarean Prevention

Cesarean/Support, Education & Concern (C/SEC)
22 Forest Road
Framingham, Massachusetts 01701
(617) 877-8266

ICAN
P.O. Box 152, University Station
Syracuse, New York 13210
(315) 424-1942

Childbearing Centers

National Association of Childbearing Centers (NACC)
RFD 1, Box 1
Perkiomenville, Pennsylvannia 18074
(215) 234-8068

Childbirth Education

Academy of Certified Childbirth Educators (ACCE)
2001 East Prairie Circle, Suite I
Olathe, Kansas 66062
(800) 444-8223
(913) 782-5116

The American Society for Psychoprophylaxis in Obstetrics (ASPO)
1840 Wilson Boulevard, Suite 204
Arlington, Virginia 22201
(800) 368-4404

Informed Homebirth/ Informed Birth and Parenting (IH)
P.O. Box 3675
Ann Arbor, Michigan 48106
(313) 662-6857

International Childbirth Education Association (ICEA)
P.O. Box 20048
Minneapolis, Minnesota 55420
(612) 854-8660

Cleft Lip, Cleft Palate

Cleft Palate Foundation
1218 Grandview Avenue
Pittsburgh, Pennsylvania 15211
(412) 481-1376
(800) 242-5338

Coping With Loss

AMEND
4324 Berrywick Terrace
St. Louis, Missouri 63128
(314) 487-7582

Compassionate Friends
Box 3696
Oak Brook, Illinois 60522-3696
(312) 990-0010

National SIDS Alliance
10500 Little Patuxent Parkway, Suite 420
Columbia, Maryland 21044
(800) 221-SIDS

National Sudden Infant Death Syndrome
501 Greensboro Drive, Suite 600
McLean, Virginia 22102
(703) 821-8955

Resolve Through Sharing
LaCrosse Lutheran Hospital
1910 South Avenue
LaCrosse, Wisconsin 54601
(608) 785-0530

Share
St. Elizabeth's Hospital
211 South Third Street
Belleville, Illinois 62222
(618) 234-2415

Cystic Fibrosis

Cystic Fibrosis Foundation
718 Arch Street, Suite 300-S
Philadelphia, Pennsylvania 19106
(215) 238-8500
(800) 344-4823

Deaf and Hearing Impaired

American Speech, Language, Hearing Association
10801 Rockville Pike
Rockville, Maryland 20852
(800) 638-8255

Better Hearing Institute
Hearing Helpline (800) 424-8576

National Association for Hearing & Speech Action
(800) 638-TALK

Down's Syndrome

National Down's Syndrome Congress
1800 Dempster Street
Park Ridge, Illinois 60068
(800) 232-NDSC

National Down's Syndrome Society
666 Broadway, Suite 810
New York, New York 10012
(800) 221-4602

Epilepsy

Epilepsy Foundation of America
4351 Garden City Drive
Landover, Maryland 20785
(301) 459-3700

Genetic Disorders

Alliance of Genetic Support Groups
1001 22nd Street NE, Suite 800
Washington, D.C. 20037
(202) 331-0942
(800) 336-GENE

National Information Center for Orphan Drugs and Rare Diseases
Box 1133
Washington, D.C. 20013
(800) 456-3505

National Organization for Rare Disorders
Box 8923
New Fairfield, Connecticut 06812
(203) 746-6518

Support for Trisomy 13/18 and Disorders
21 Ryers Avenue
Cheltenham, Pennsylvania 19102
(215) 663-9652

Tay Sachs National & Allied Diseases, Inc.
422 Lincoln Avenue
Highland Park, New Jersey 08904
(201) 246-8080

Handicapped Children

Council for Exceptional Children
1920 Association Drive
Reston, Virginia 22091
(703) 620-3660

National Information Center for Children With Handicaps
Box 1492
Washington, D.C. 20013
(703) 893-6061
(800) 999-5599

Heart Defects

American Heart Association
121 South Broad Street
Philadelphia, Pennsylvania 19107
(215) 735-3865

Congenital Heart Information Program
Box 15131
Baton Rouge, Louisiana 70815
(504) 928-1458

Heartline
10500 Noland Road
Overland Park, Kansas 66215
(913) 492-6317

Mended Hearts
7320 Greenville Avenue
Dallas, Texas 75231
(214) 750-5442

High-Risk Pregnancy

Parent Care, Inc.
101½ South Union
Alexandria, Virginia 22314-3323
(703) 836-4678

Homeopathy

For complete catalogues of homeopathic products:
Standard Homeopathic Company
Box 61067
Los Angeles, California 90061
(215) 520-0580
(800) 624-9659

Hydrocephalus

National Hydrocephalus Foundation
22427 South River Road
Joliet, Illinois 60436
(815) 467-6548

Medical Organizations

American Academy of Pediatrics
Box 927
141 NW Point Boulevard
Elk Grove Village, Illinois 60009-0927
(312) 228-5005

American College of OB/GYN
409 12th Street SW
Washington, D.C. 20024-2188
(800) 673-8444

American Fertility Society
2140 11th Avenue South, Suite 200
Birmingham, Alabama 35205-2800
(205) 933-8494

Mental Retardation

Association for Retarded Citizens
500 East Border Street, Suite 300
Arlington, Texas 76010
(800) 433-5255

Spina Bifida

Spina Bifida Association
4590 MacArthur Boulevard NW, Suite 250
Washington, DC 20007
(800) 621-3141

Twins

Twinline
Box 10066
Berkeley, California 94709
(415) 644-8063

Bibliography

Amniotomy

Baumgarten, K. 1976. Advantages and disadvantages of low amniotomy. *Journal of Perinatal Medicine* 4:3–11.

Caldeyro-Barcia, R., et al. 1974. Adverse perinatal effects of early amniotomy during labor. In *Modern Perinatal Medicine*, ed. L. Gluck. Chicago: Year Book Medical Publishers.

Friedman, E., and M. Sachtelben. 1963. Amniotomy and the course of labor. *Obstetrics and Gynecology* 22: 755–70.

Kubli, F. 1968. Influence of labor on fetal acid-base balance. *Clinical Obstetrics and Gynecology* 2: 168–91.

Lumley, J., and C. Wood. 1971. Transient fetal acidosis and artificial rupture of the membranes, *Australia–New Zealand* Journal of Obstetrics and Gynecology. 2: 221–25.

Lynaugh, K. H. The effects of early elective amniotomy on the length of labor and the condition of the fetus. *Journal of Nurse-Midwifery*. Vol. 1, 1989

Analgesics

Myers, R. E. 1970. Use of sedatives, analgesics, and anesthetic drugs during labor and delivery: Bane or boon? *American Journal of Obstetrics and Gynecology* 133, No. 1 (January): 83–104.

Anesthesia, Regional

Ralston, D. H., and S. M. Schnider. 1978. The fetal and neonatal effects of regional anesthesia in obstetrics. *Anesthesiology* 48, No. 1 (January): 34–64.

Cesarean Surgery and Cesarean Prevention

Caire, J. 1978. Are current rates of cesarean justified? *Southern Medical Journal* 71, No. 5 (May)

Gilstrap, L., J. Hauth, and S. Toussaint. 1984. Cesarean section: Changing incidence and indications. *Obstetrics and Gynecology* 63, No. 2 (February)

Minkoff, H., and R. Schwartz. 1980. The rising cesarean section rate: Can it safely be reversed? *Obstetrics and Gynecology* 56, No. 2 (August)

Childbearing Center Birth

Daniels, S. 1979. *Birth and the Family Journal* 6, No. 4 (Winter): 259–66.

Faison, J. B., et al. 1979. The childbearing center: an alternative birth setting. *Obstetrics and Gynecology* 54, No. 4 (October)

Lubic, R. W. The rise of the birth center alternative. *The Nation's Health* 7. 1983.

Ostrowsky, L. L. 1982. *Alternative birth centers*. Berkeley: California Department of Health Services.

Reinke, C. 1982. Outcomes of the first 527 births at the Birthplace in Seattle. *Birth* 9, No. 4 (Winter) 238.

Sculphome, A., A. G. McLeod, and E. G. Robertson, A birth center affiliated with the tertiary care center: comparison of outcome. *Obstetrics and Gynecology* 67, No. 4 (April) 598–603.

Electronic Fetal Monitoring

National Institutes of Health. 1979. *Antenatal diagnostics*. Publication no. 79-1973 (April). Bethesda, Md.

Friedman, E. A. 1986. The obstetrician's dilemma: How much fetal monitoring and cesarean section is enough? *New England Journal of Medicine* 315, No. 10: 641–43.

Haverkamp, A., et al. 1976. The evaluation of continuous fetal heart rate monitoring in high-risk pregnancy. *American Journal of Obstetrics and Gynecology* 1, No. 3 (June)

Haverkamp, A. 1979. Does anyone need fetal monitors? In *Compulsory hospitalization*, vol. 1, ed. Stewart and Stewart, 137. Marble Hill, Mo.: NAPSAC Publications.

Kelso, I., et al. 1978. An assessment of continuous fetal heart rate monitoring in labor. *American Journal of Obstetrics and Gynecology* 131, No. 5, 526–32.

Paul, R., J. Huey, and C. Yeager. 1977. Clinical fetal monitoring: Its effect on cesarean section rate and perinatal mortality: Five-year trends. *Postgraduate Medicine* 61: 160.

Shy, K. K., et al. 1990. Effects of electronic fetal-heart-rate monitoring as compared with periodic auscultation on the neurologic development of premature infants. *New England Journal of Medicine*, March 1, 1990.

Episiotomy

Banta, D., and S. Thacker. 1982. The risks and benefits of episiotomy: A review. *Birth* 9, No. 1 (Spring)

Fathers and Breastfeeding

Jordan, P. L., and V. R. 1990. Wall. Breastfeeding and fathers: Illuminating the darker side. *Birth* 17, No. 4 (December): 210–13.

Jordan, P. L. 1986. Breastfeeding as a risk factor for fathers. *Journal of Gynecological and Neonatal Nursing* (March/April): 94–97.

Waletzy, L. R., 1979. Husbands' problems with breastfeeding. *American Journal of Orthopsychiatry* 49: 349–52.

Home Birth

American College of Obstetricians and Gynecologists. 1978. Health department data shows danger of home births. January 4, 1978.

Burnett, C., et al. Home delivery and neonatal mortality in North Carolina. *Journal of the American Medical Association* 244, No. 24: 2741–45.

Kitzinger, S., and David, eds. 1978. *The place of birth.* New York: Oxford University Press.

Hazell, L. 1975. A study of 300 elective home births. *Birth and the Family Journal* 2: 11–18.

Hinds, M., et al. Neonatal outcomes in planned v. unplanned out-of-hospital births in Kentucky. *Journal of the American Medical Association* 253, No. 85: 1578–82.

Hosford, E. 1978. The home birth movement. *Journal of Nurse-Midwifery* 21, No. 3 (Fall) 29–30.

Sagov, S., et al. 1984. *Home birth: A practitioner's guide to birth outside the hospital.* Rockland, Md.: Aspen Systems Corp.

Searles, C. 1985. The impetus toward home birth. *Journal of Nurse-Midwifery* 26: 51–56.

Shy, K., F. Frost, and J. Ullom. 1980. Out-of-hospital delivery in Washington State, 1975–1977. *American Journal of Obstetrics and Gynecology* 137: 547–52.

Sullivan, D. A., and R. Weitz. 1988. *Labor pains: modern midwives and home birth.* New Haven: Yale University Press.

Homeopathy and Labor

Day, C. E. I. 1984. Control of stillbirths in pigs using homeopathy. *British Homeopathic Journal* 73 (July): 142–43.

Hospital Alternatives

DeVries, R. 1983. Image and reality: an evaluation of hospital alternative birth centers. *Journal of Nurse-Midwifery* 28: 3–9.

Williams, J. K., and M. R. Mervis. 1990. Use of the labor-delivery-recovery room in an urban tertiary care hospital. *American Journal of Obstetrics and Gynecology* 162: 23–24.

Waryas, F. S., and M. B. Luebbers. 1986. A cluster system for maternity care. *Maternal-Child Nursing* 2: 98–100.

McKay S., and C. R. Phillips. 1984. *Family centered maternity care.* Rockville, Md.: Aspen Systems Corp.

Induction of Labor

Calder, A. A., et al. 1974. Increased bilirubin levels in neonates after induction of labor by intravenous prostaglandin or oxytocin. *Lancet* 2: 1339–42.

Oski, F. A. 1975. Oxytocin and hyperbilirubinemia. *American Journal of Disabled Child* 129: 1139–40.

Wingerup, L., and G. Ekman. Local application of prostaglandin E2 for cervical ripening or induction of term labor. *Clinical Obstetrics and Gynecology* 7, No. 1: 95–105.

Labor Support

Bennett A., et al. 1985. Antenatal preparation and labor support in relation to birth outcomes. *Birth* 12, No. 1 (Spring): 9–15

Birch, E. R. 1986. The experience of therapeutic touch received during labor. *Journal of Nurse-Midwifery* 31, No. 6 (November/December): 270–76.

Bowes, W. 1992. Labor support: many unanswered questions remain. *Birth* 19, No. 1 (March): 38–39.

Copstick, S. M., et al. Partner support and the use of coping techniques in labor. *Journal of Psychosomatic Research* 30, No. 4: 497–503.

Hofmeyr, J. G., et al. Companionship to modify the clinical birth environment: Effects on progress and perceptions of labour, and breastfeeding. *British Journal of Obstetrics and Gynecology* 98, No. 756: 162–64.

Hommel, F. 1969. Natural childbirth—nurses in private practice as monitrice. *American Journal of Nursing* 69, No. 7 (July): 1446–50.

Kennell, J., et al. 1991. Continuous emotional support during labor in a U.S. hospital. *Journal of the American Medical Association* 265, No. 17 (May): 2197–2201.

Kennell, J. H. 1982. The physiologic effects of a supportive companion (doula) during labor. In *Birth, interaction, and attachment*, Silkman, N.J.: Johnson and Johnson.

Klaus, M. H., et al. 1986. Effects of social support during parturition on maternal and infant morbidity. *British Medical Journal* 293, No. 6547 (September): 585–87.

McNiven, P., et al. 1992. Supporting women in labor: A work sampling of the activities of labor and delivery nurses. *Birth* 19, No. 1 (March): 3–8

Mercer, R. T., K. C. Hackley, and A. G. Bostrom. Relationship of psychosocial and perinatal variables to perception of childbirth. *Nursing Research* 32, No. 4 (July/August): 202–207.

Sosa, R., J. Kennell, and M. Klaus. The effect of a supportive companion on perinatal problems, length of labor, and mother-infant interaction. *New England Journal of Medicine* 303, No. 11 (September): 597–600.

Maternal Position in Labor

Caldeyro-Barcia, R. 1975. Supine called worst position during labor and delivery. *Obstetrics and Gynecology News* (June) 101

Liu, Y. 1979. Position during labor and delivery: history and perspective. *Journal of Nurse-Midwifery* 24, No. 3 (May/June)

Naroll, F., R. Naroll, and F. H. Howard. 1961. Position of women in childbirth: A study in data quality control. *American Journal of Obstetrics and Gynecology* 82: 943–54.

Roberts, J. 1980: Alternative positions for childbirth, part I: first stage of labor. Part II: second stage of labor. *Journal of Nurse-Midwifery* 25: 11–30.

Russell, J. 1982. The rationale of primitive delivery positions. *British Journal of Obstetrics and Gynecology* 89: 712–15.

Midwifery

Gaskin, I. M. 1978. *Spiritual midwifery.* Summertown, Tenn.: The Book Publishing Company.

Hosford, E. 1976. Alternative patterns of nurse-midwifery care. *Journal of Nurse-Midwifery* 21, No.3: 28.

Mehl, L. et al. 1980. Evaluation of outcomes of non-nurse midwives: Matched comparisons with physicians. *Women and Health* 5: 17–29.

Montgomery, T. 1981. A case for nurse-midwives. *American Journal of Obstetrics* 109: 50–58.

Varney, H. 1980. *Nurse-midwifery.* Boston: Blackwell Scientific Publications.

Mind, Emotions, and Labor

Lederman, R. P., et al. 1979. "Comparison of prostaglandin E2 and intravenous oxytocin for induction of labor." Obstetrics and Gynecology 54: 581.

Newton, N. 1982. *Maternal emotions.* New York: Paul B. Hoeber.

———, 1977. The effect of fear and disturbance in labor. In *Twenty-first Century Obstetrics Now,* ed. Stewart and Stewart, 62–71. Marble Hill, Mo.: NAPSAC Publications.

Miscellaneous

Carr, K. C. 1980. Obstetric practices which protect against neonatal morbidity: Focus on maternal position in labor and birth. *Birth* 7, No. 4 (Winter): 249–54.

Dyson, D. C., et al. 1986. Antepartum external cephalic version under tocolysis. *Obstetrics and Gynecology* 67, No. 1: 63–68.

Sonstegard, L. J. 1981. Rotating the malpositioned fetus. *Perinatal Press* 5, No. 5 (June).

Parent-Infant Attachment

Barnet, C. R., et al. 1970. Neonatal separation: The maternal side of interactional deprivation. *Pediatrics* 54: 197.

Klaus, M. H., and J. H. Kennel. 1976. *Maternal-infant bonding: The impact of early separation or loss on family development.* St. Louis: C. V. Mosby.

Klaus, M., and J. Kennell. 1970. Mothers separated from their newborn infants. *Pediatric Clinics of North America* 17: 1015–37.

Perineal Shaving

Kantor, H, et al. 1965. Value of shaving the pudendal-perineal area in delivery preparation. *Obstetrics and Gynecology* 25: 509–12.

Postpartum Support

Raphael, D. 1981. The midwife as doula: A guide to mothering the mother. *Journal of Nurse-Midwifery* 26, No. 6 (November/December): 13–15.

Prenatal Nutrition

S. Taffel. 1986. Maternal weight gain and the outcome of pregnancy, United States, 1980. *Vital and Health Statistics,* series 21, no. 44, DHHS Publication No. 86-1922. National Center for Health Statistics. Public Health Service. Washington, D.C.: U.S. Government Printing Office (June)

Psychology of Pregnancy: Fathers

Jordan, P. L. 1990. Laboring for relevance: expectant and new fatherhood. *Nursing Research* 39, No. 1: 11–16.

May, K. A. 1980. A typology of detachment/involvement styles adopted during pregnancy by first-time fathers. *Western Journal of Nursing Research* 2: 445–61.

May, K. A. 1982. The father as observer. *Maternal-Child Nursing* 7: 319–22.

———. Three phases of father involvement in pregnancy. *Nursing Research* 31: 337–42.

———. 1982. Factors contributing to first-time fathers' readiness for fatherhood. *Family Relations* 31: 353–62.

Psychology of Pregnancy: Mothers

Lederman, R. P. 1984. *Psychosocial adaptation in pregnancy.* Englewood Cliffs, N.J: Prentice-Hall.

Macfarlane, A. 1978. *The psychology of childbirth*. Cambridge, Mass.: Harvard University Press.

Mercer, R. T. 1986. *First-time motherhood*. New York: Springer.

Rubin, R. 1984. *Maternal identity and the maternal experience*. New York: Springer.

Waterbirth

Church, Linda. 1989. *Journal of Nurse-Midwifery* 34, No.4 (July/August) 168.

Index